THROUGH THE FOG

A Guide to Caring for Loved Ones with Mental Illness

by
Leah DeMarest

THROUGH THE FOG

A Guide to Caring for Loved Ones with Mental Illness

Table of Contents

Introduction

Helping a loved one navigate the choppy seas of mental illness is both a privilege and a challenge. This book aims to provide you with a strong understanding of mental illnesses and how to best support those in your life who may be suffering. Whether you're still coming to terms with a close one's diagnosis or you're knee-deep in the daily turmoil, this book beckons you into a world where empathy, understanding and open communication take center stage in creating an atmosphere conducive to recovery and support.

Many can attest to the fact that mental illness is shrouded in mystery and marred by stigma. This introduction seeks to demystify the concept, shedding light on what mental illnesses are and aren't. You see, far too often, people struggle under the weight of misinformation, bias, and stereotypes-our goal is to dispel those erroneous beliefs and land on a more compassionate and informed footing. Knowledge is our primary weapon, and it's upon us to wield it with finesse and purpose.

Recognizing that every journey is unique, this book does not prescribe a one-size-fits-all approach to supporting a loved one living with a mental illness. Instead, it is crafted to serve as a guide, an ally in navigating the often unseen and misunderstood aspects of mental disorders. It aims to encourage dialogue between you and your loved ones, to construct bridges where walls previously stood, and to foster an environment of mutual trust, understanding, and collaboration.

The chapters that follow are designed to gently lead you through the maze of mental health, debunking myths, exposing truths, and equipping you with practical advice along the way. They delve into the realms of stigma, communication, caregiving, crisis management, and legal considerations, providing you with a comprehensive understanding, and, more importantly, actionable strategies to apply in your unique situation.

The first chapter commences our journey by presenting an overview of mental illness, imparting critical knowledge about its complexities and nuances. By instilling a clear-cut understanding of the landscape at hand, it sets you up for informed engagement and interaction with your loved one.

Proceeding to the second chapter, it shines a light on the dark recesses of stigma and prejudice embedded in our society's fabric. Armed with this knowledge, you're better positioned to counteract these damaging beliefs, ultimately contributing to a holistic advocacy for mental health.

Chapters three and four focus intensely on communication—how to encourage your loved one to seek help and how to effectively convey empathy, concern, and support. Here, you're exposed to the techniques essential to fostering meaningful dialogue, tearing down walls, and building bridges of understanding and connection.

The following chapters explore the depths of the caregiver's role, defining proactive steps you can take to help your loved one. From dispensing prescribed medications to providing emotional support and navigating the job market, these chapters are designed to equip you with practical, hands-on advice for day-to-day living.

Chapter six unwraps the elements of a positive relationship. Filled with tips about setting healthy boundaries, practicing empathy, and fostering mutual respect and trust, this chapter aims to enlighten you on the art of nurturing a supportive and uplifting environment.

Crisis management, an often disconcerting aspect of mental health care, is the focus of the seventh chapter. By providing you with knowledge on recognizing signs of crises and how to effectively respond, this section nurtures your ability to navigate emergency situations with calm and wisdom.

Chapter eight delves into the crucial aspects of legal and financial planning, guiding you to prepare for long-term care. Here, you gain a vantage point on how to ensure the protection of your loved one's rights and financial security.

Chapter nine places essential emphasis on the importance of self-care for caregivers. Throughout this book, you're acknowledged not just as a caregiver, but as an individual, with your wellbeing integral to the overall journey. This chapter avails you with a myriad of self-care techniques, highlighting its importance in the entire caregiving process.

Finally, the last chapter guides you towards essential resources and support that can supplement your stewardship role in your loved one's mental health journey. From mental health professionals and clinics to support groups for caregivers and online resources, this chapter underscores that you are not alone on this journey.

So, as you turn these pages, remember that you are not alone. This book becomes your companion, your guide, your counsel in navigating through the labyrinth that can be mental illness. It is a journey of discovery, of understanding, and most importantly, of love. Because when you love someone, you want to walk with them even in the darkest paths, even when every step is a stumbling block. This book equips you with the tools, resources, and wisdom to lovingly and effectively support your loved one.

Chapter 1:
Understanding Mental Illness

Comprehending mental illness requires more than just a basic knowledge of symptoms or diagnoses. Instead, it involves understanding the complex interplay between biology, psychology, and the environment which leads to these conditions. This chapter aims to help you grasp the diverse and multifaceted nature of mental illness.

At the heart of understanding mental illness is the recognition that these conditions are legitimate and serious, affecting a person's thoughts, emotions, and behaviors. Mental illnesses can disrupt a person's ability to function in daily life, form relationships and maintain employment. They aren't a sign of a lack of discipline or moral failing but are genuine medical conditions.

Everything from mood disorders, anxiety disorders, eating disorders, to bipolar disorder, schizophrenia, and post-traumatic stress disorder falls under the umbrella of mental illness. One critical aspect to appreciate is that mental illnesses vary greatly. Each has its own set of symptoms, causes, and effects, making them as diverse as their sufferers; and each person experiences their diagnosis differently than the next. For example, Jim and John may both be diagnosed with depression, but Jim may experience feelings of guilt, excessive hunger, insomnia, excessive crying, and thoughts of suicide; but John, with the same diagnosis, may experience apathy, hopelessness, excessive sleepiness, loss of appetite, social isolation, agitation and irritability.

The Biological Aspect

In many cases, mental illnesses are rooted in biology. Some people inherit genes from their parents that make them more susceptible to certain conditions; they may be born with an overactive Brodmann area of the brain, or born with a unique pattern of epigenetic tags in the brain, or their brain might naturally produce too much or too little of a certain chemicals in the brain called neurotransmitters. These predispositions can lead to the development of a mental illness when paired with environmental triggers or stressful life events.

The Psychological Aspect

The core of many mental illnesses lies in the realm of psychology. Unresolved trauma, feelings, and emotions can give rise to various psychological disorders. Some examples of psychological aspects are abuse, neglect, or a major loss or death of a close loved one. It's vital not to oversimplify mental illness as merely an emotional problem. These conditions are much more complex and multi-layered.

The Environmental Aspect

On top of biological and psychological factors, environmental elements often significantly contribute to mental illness. Traumatic life experiences, high stress levels, exposure to violence, neglect or abuse, can all contribute to the development of these conditions.

Another crucial point to understand is that anyone can be affected by mental illness, regardless of their age, gender, social status, or ethnicity. There's no immunity to mental health issues, and they don't indicate any failure or weakness in a person.

Rather than seeing people with mental illness as "other," it's vital to remember they are people first and foremost. A mental illness is just one aspect of their identity and experience, not the totality of who they are.

Also, mental illnesses can be chronic or episodic. Some may have one episode and never have another, while others may have recurring episodes or symptoms that persist over time. The course and effects of mental illness can vary significantly from person to person.

It's also critical to know that people with mental illnesses can recover or manage their symptoms effectively. A combination of medication, therapy, lifestyle changes, and support from others can make a significant difference. Such recovery doesn't necessarily mean the total absence of symptoms, but improved ability to function and a better quality of life. Though, many people do live with lifelong mental illness and without proper treatment their symptoms can intensify and worsen with age.

A common misconception is that people with mental illness are violent or unpredictable. However, the vast majority of individuals with mental health issues are no more likely to be violent than anyone else. They are, in fact, more likely to be victims of violence themselves. People with mental illness are your neighbors, teachers, hair stylists, doctors, waitresses, therapists, dog groomers, dieticians, etc. The vast majority of people with a diagnosed mental illness are very successful people, based off of societal norms for success.

The stigma around mental illness can often be more challenging than the illness itself. It can lead to isolation, discrimination, and a reluctance to seek help. Understanding mental illness is fundamental to combating this stigma and being an effective supporter and caregiver for your loved one.

Comprehension of mental illness is only a starting point, but it's one that can lead to empathy and improved connection with a loved one dealing with such conditions. Understanding the realities of mental illness can assist in breaking down stigma, fostering open communication, and starting the path towards support and potential recovery.

Mental Illness Stigma

Having traversed the terrain of understanding mental illness in the previous section, we now wade into a sensitive and often misunderstood topic-stigma associated with mental illness. Despite advancements in our collective societal understanding of mental health, stigma remains a prevalent and persistent issue. It's seen in many forms-from inadvertent remarks at dinner tables to more institutionalized prejudices.

Stigma can be broadly categorized into two types: social stigma and self-stigma. Social stigma refers to the prejudiced attitudes others have about mental illness while self-stigma is the internalizing of these negative stereotypes and prejudices by individuals with a mental illness.

Social stigma manifests in various ways. It's not uncommon to encounter people who harbor biases and misconceptions. They may, for instance, view mental illness as a character flaw or sign of weakness. Outdated and unhelpful beliefs perpetuate these stereotypes, leading to discrimination, reluctance to seek help, and delayed treatment for those affected.

Self-stigma, on the other hand, is intimately related to an individual's self-worth and self-esteem. When someone with a mental illness internalizes societal prejudices, they may begin to believe that they are somehow less valuable than others. This can lead to feelings of shame and worthlessness, and can substantially derail the healing and recovery process.

It's crucial to understand that stigma isn't just harmful because it's hurtful-it has tangible, real-life consequences. Most notably, it discourages individuals from seeking help. Avoidance of treatment due to the fear of being labelled 'mentally ill' or 'unstable' can exacerbate the ailment, making recovery more complex and long-drawn.

Furthermore, stigma can pervade all spheres of life, impacting relationships, education, and employment opportunities. Relationships can be strained as loved ones may struggle to understand the condition, leading to social isolation of the individual. Education and employment opportunities can be compromised due to perceived instability or unpredictability.

So, what reinforces this stigma? One of the primary culprits is misinformation and lack of education about mental health. Mental illness is often misunderstood, leading to fear and exclusion of those affected. Simplistic and generalized media portrayals add to misconceptions, painting affected individuals as dangerous, unpredictable outcasts.

In the face of such widespread bias, it's important to remember the power of education in breaking down these barriers. Real, on-the-ground awareness can help challenge stereotypes and debunk myths perpetuating stigma. Education isn't just about imparting facts, it's also about fostering empathy by helping people understand the human side of living with mental illness.

Stigma can be fought at an institutional level too. Legal protections against discrimination for people with mental illnesses can go a long way in creating an equitable environment. Further, schools, employers, and policy makers can institute initiatives that promote understanding, acceptance, and support for mental health issues.

It's also important to tackle self-stigma. One potential approach lies in empowerment. Encouraging those with mental illness to speak up about their experiences can be cathartic and further societal understanding. In addition, support groups can provide a safe space for people to share, learn, and gain validation of their experiences.

Stigma is not an insurmountable wall, it's a series of misconceptions that can, over time, be dismantled through understanding and compassion. As you move forth on this journey of support and connect with your loved ones, it's crucial to be mindful of the biases you may harbor and instead, approach mental illness with kindness, empathy, and respect.

Understanding the fact that seeking help isn't a sign of weakness but courage can also contribute towards combating stigma. Mental illness is a part of the human experience; it doesn't reflect poorly on the one struggling, rather it underscores their resilience in the face of adversity.

Stigma doesn't only compromise societal perception but also personal self-esteem and sense of self-worth. It creates barriers to seeking help, accessing opportunities, forming relationships, and living a fulfilling life. Misinformation promotes stigma which can be dismantled through education, equitable policies, and gradual societal shift in attitudes. Dealing effectively with mental illness requires us to not only confront the illness itself, but also the attitudes, beliefs, and stereotypes we associate with it.

<u>Chapter 1 Key Take Aways</u>

1. Mental illness is diverse and multifaceted with a complex interplay between biology, psychology, and environment.

2. Anyone can be affected by mental illness, regardless of age, gender, social status, or ethnicity.

3. Understanding mental illness is fundamental in combating mental illness stigma.

Chapter 2:
Encouraging a Loved One to Seek Help

As we've previously delved into the essential groundwork of mental illness understanding and stigma dismantling, it's now time to step into the delicate terrain of encouraging your loved one to seek professional assistance. This chapter is about the pivotal yet sensitive act of initiating the conversation around mental health. It is necessary to approach this with a blend of humility, love, and unwavering patience, always mindful of the tender tendrils of trust that need to be nurtured. While the first step is expressing your concerns, it is essential to remember that responding to resistance and denials is a part of the process and requires care. Denials and resistance can come in varied forms, sometimes blatant, sometimes veiled in avoidance. Standing at this juncture, act not with force but with quiescent determination, underlining the fact that the impetus to seek help is not indicative of weakness, rather it's about the courage to embark on a journey towards healing and wellbeing. The talks you have today, the space you hold, has the potential to bring about life-altering transformations tomorrow.

Initiate the Conversation

Addressing loved ones' mental health issues may feel intimidating. It's normal to fear potentially triggering fragile emotions or eliciting defensive reactions. Yet, communication is crucial in setting foundations for their healing journey.

Conversations about mental health break the ice, unveiling the tools and supports needed for recovery.

The first step is to prepare yourself. Understand that this conversation might be challenging, both for you and your loved one. It's important to approach it with sensitivity, empathy, and patience. Be prepared for denial, defense mechanisms, or even anger. These reactions are common and often indicative of a person's internal struggle.

Before you begin the conversation, it's helpful to gather your thoughts first. This involves carefully reflecting upon the observations and concerns that led you to believe your loved one might be struggling with their mental health. It may also be advantageous to practice expressing these thoughts aloud, either to yourself or with a trusted friend or advisor.

When you're ready to initiate the conversation, make sure you choose the right time and place. You'll want an environment that is comfortable and private, free from distractions. Above all, ensure the place is safe to discuss personal matters openly and honestly. Timing also plays a key role. Choose a moment when they are relatively calm and receptive, not during a peak of anxiety or distress.

Begin the conversation with transparency. Convey love, concern, and the intent behind your words. Make clear that you're not trying to point out flaws or criticize them, but rather express concern out of love and the desire to understand their experience. Start with phrases like "I've noticed" or "I'm worried" rather than making any outright judgments or declarations.

Remember to keep your tone calm and non-judgmental. Acknowledge that the individual's feelings are valid and reassure them that you're there as a supportive and understanding figure, not as an interrogator. You're seeking insight into their experience-not trying to diagnose or offer unsolicited advice.

Encourage self-expression from them, too. Ask open-ended questions to allow them to share their feelings and experiences. Be patient and don't rush them to answer. Your role here is to listen and create an environment where they are comfortable expressing themselves.

While discussing it, make sure you emphasize their strengths. Use concrete examples of their resilience and remind them of times when they've overcome previous challenges. This recognizes their abilities and instills hope for recovery with positive reinforcement.

Shun assertive phrases like "you must" or "you should". Instead, use supportive language like "you might find it helpful" or "consider the benefits of". This gives them autonomy over their decision-making, reducing defensive reactions.

Touch upon the benefits of professional mental health treatment in your conversation. Instead of placing an expectation, present it as a beneficial choice. Because, in the end, they're the one who will decide their course of action.

Always remember to normalize the conversation around mental health. Use day-to-day examples or instances to remove stigma and induce comfort in discussing their feelings.

Expect various reactions without assuming a negative one. They may react with acceptance, denial, anger, or even relief. At this juncture, aim to maintain a comforting presence, offering reassurances that these feelings are normal.

Finally, ensure to end the conversation on a positive note. Remind them of your constant support and convey hope about the potential for recovery. Reinforce that seeking help isn't a sign of weakness, but rather an act of courage.

Initiating conversations about mental health might be tough, but it's a vital stepping stone in the journey towards support and understanding. By fostering a compassionate dialogue, you could help your loved one break the barrier of silence, navigate through their struggles, and stride forward on their road to recovery.

Overcoming Resistance and Denials

Encouraging a loved one with mental illness to seek assistance can be a tremendous challenge, particularly when they're resistant or in denial about their condition. It's essential to approach the situation with patience, sensitivity, and understanding, knowing that acceptance is often the first major hurdle in the journey toward mental health.

Resistance and denial often stem from fear or misunderstandings about mental illness. Stigma plays a significant role here, with loved ones fearing judgement or criticism from others. It could also be because the thought of tackling their mental health issues feels too overwhelming, or they don't believe they need help at all.

Here's where you may start to feel powerless, but it's important to remember that you have a critical role in helping your loved one navigate these waters. And you can adopt several strategies to assist your loved one in overcoming resistance and denials.

It's crucial to show them that you're on their side. Speak from a place of genuine care and concern, expressing that you want to ease their pain and improve their quality of life. Ensure them they are not alone in their journey, and that seeking help is a sign of strength, not weakness.

Education plays a significant part in breaking down these barriers. It can be useful for you and your loved one to learn together about mental health. This education helps to destigmatize mental illness and shed light on the reality that it is a common human experience and not a personal failing. You can use various resources like reading materials, support groups, online resources, or even professional consultations.

Additionally, it's helpful to provide tangible examples of how seeking help can benefit them; real-life stories of others who've sought help and experienced healing can be powerful proof that things can get better. Focus on their ability to regain control and function, emphasizing the potential for them to find joy and satisfaction in life again.

Highlighting the confidentiality of seeking professional help can also mitigate fear. Mental health professionals are bound by stringent privacy laws and ethics, ensuring safe spaces to express emotions and fears without judgement.

Unfortunately, denial can be deeply ingrained, and you might not see progress after the first, second or even third conversation. It's critical here to remain patient and persistent, consistently conveying love and concern without pushing too hard or being overly aggressive. It may be frustrating, but remember that change often takes time.

If your loved one continues to resist or deny the need for help, consider seeking advice from a mental health professional yourself. They can provide guidance on ways to approach the situation and strategies to use, as well as provide you with support during this challenging time.

An intervention may be beneficial in certain situations, but this should only be done under the guidance of a mental health professional. A sudden, forced confrontation could backfire, establishing further resistance or even damaging the relationship.

There might also be the need to involve other individuals, but choose carefully. Select people who carry the same message of care, concern, and desire to support healing. High-emotion situations can inadvertently escalate if not carefully managed.

However, it's crucial to be prepared for the possibility that your loved one may still refuse help. In this situation, establishing boundaries to protect your own mental health becomes paramount. You cannot force someone to accept help, and it's important to acknowledge that your loved one has a right to make decisions about their treatment.

Finally, make sure to take care of your mental health. Understand that it's okay to feel overwhelmed and consider reaching out for help or joining a support group. You're doing your best, and that's more than enough.

In this journey of overcoming resistance and denial, patience, persistence and plenty of empathy are key. Remember, lasting change takes time but with love, understanding, and the right support, the road to improved and consistent mental health is attainable.

Chapter 2 Key Take Aways

1. Communication is crucial in setting foundations for the healing journey and vital for you to give the appropriate support and understanding that your loved one needs.

2. It is important to communicate with sensitivity, empathy, and patience.

3. Be prepared for denial, defense mechanisms, anger, resistance, and the unexpected.

4. Educating yourself on mental illness and obtaining your own support from a therapist can be crucial for your role as a caregiver.

Chapter 3:
Effective Communication Strategies

Now that we've broached the subject of help with your loved one, it's essential you arm yourself with the right tools to have effective conversations. One of the most potent tools at your disposal is communication. When it comes to mental illness, the significance of communication cannot be overstated. It isn't just about what you say, but how you say it, how well you listen, and the non-verbal cues you convey. At first, recognizing and breaking through the barriers hindering communication will require patience and insight. However, once identified, these obstacles can be turned into bridges of understanding. Exercising active listening, for instance, will not just make your loved one feel heard, but also valued and understood. When you actively listen, you're not just waiting for your turn to speak; you're hearing, absorbing, and responding to the emotions behind the words. Remember, communication isn't solely about the words we use. Non-verbal cues often carry as much weight as words. Things like eye contact, touch, and tone can often express what words fail to capture. Mastering these strategies will help establish a two-way street of empathy and understanding, fostering a supportive environment in the face of mental illness.

Understanding the Barrier

One of the key factors when trying to establish effective communication strategies with a loved one suffering from a mental illness is understanding the barriers that might exist. It is quite a journey, one in which the importance of patience and empathy cannot be understated.

Breaking it down, the barriers might be physical, psychological, or social in nature. By physical barriers, we refer to literal obstructions such as doors or walls, or more symbolically, the impairment caused by the mental illness itself. It could limit the patient's cognitive function, speech, or their ability to interpret and understand social cues.

Psychological barriers, meanwhile, are predominantly influenced by personal thoughts, feelings, and emotions. For instance, if a loved one is experiencing depression or anxiety, they might harbor feelings of uncertainty, fear, or guilt. These intense emotions might lead to the development of a defense mechanism that shields them from perceived threats-the conversation about their mental health could act as a trigger, serving to further pull the person into a protective shell.

On the societal front, the stigma around mental health becomes a formidable obstacle. When your loved one constantly fears judgment from society, they may resist any attempts of discussion or assistance in relation to their mental health. Misunderstandings, misconceptions, and general ignorance about mental illness serve to solidify this barrier, encouraging patterns of denial and evasion.

To dismantle these barriers, understanding the nature of the mental illness your loved one is dealing with is a vital step. Different illnesses are characterized by different symptoms and ways they influence a person's behavior and thinking. By educating yourself about these illnesses, you shape a more empathetic approach, demonstrating your eagerness to understand the challenges faced by your loved one.

As you address and work through these barriers, your posture and demeanor significantly influence the effectiveness of your communication efforts. You need to emit warmth and authenticity when talking to your loved ones. By doing so, you create an environment of acceptance and safety where they feel free to express their thoughts and feelings.

As important as it is to keep the line of communication open, steering clear of the pressure to talk can be beneficial. In certain cases, pressurizing someone with a mental illness to engage in a discussion about their feelings can counteract the intent of essentially showing them you care, understand, and are there for them.

Also, you'd want to avoid oversimplifying or reducing their experiences to generic cliches. Your intention might be to console or reassure, but reassuring phrases, like "everything will be alright," can often be perceived as dismissive or belittling of their emotional state. Remember, you're not there to 'fix' them, you're there to support them.

Another common barrier is the mistaken belief that an individual with mental illness is incapable of partaking in decisions about their care. This can often undermine their sense of autonomy and self-worth. It is essential to involve your loved one in these discussions, contingent on the readiness of the individual.

Understanding and acknowledging these barriers isn't the same as accepting them as intractable obstacles. It's seeing them for what they are–formidable, yet not insurmountable. This perspective is what ultimately empowers us to break down the walls of fear, stigma, and misunderstanding, paving the way towards compassionate and effective communication.

Remember, you can't always pre-empt or prepare for every barrier you might face. Sometimes, unexpected challenges may arise, and that's alright. What's key is having a general understanding of probable obstacles and holding onto the willingness to adapt your approach as needed.

Do bear in mind that the journey won't always be smooth, the conversation may meander, uncomfortable silences might arise, and these are all significant parts of the process. Don't shun these moments. Instead, take them as opportunities to learn, adapt, and evolve in your communication approach.

In navigating these barriers, it might help to remember that while you are learning to understand your loved one's new reality, they are also trying to come to terms with their experiences. Empathy, love, and patience are essential in ensuring open and effective communication processes.

Understanding the barriers to communication doesn't make you responsible for removing them all. Sometimes, it's about knowing when to seek professional help for your loved one. This need for help shouldn't be viewed as a failing but as a strength, accepting that some barriers are beyond your capacity to handle but within reach of skilled professionals committed to mental wellness.

By understanding the barriers in communication, you deepen your insight into your loved one's lived experiences. You forge a stronger connection with them, fostering trust and openness that forms the backbone of any successful communication strategy.

Active Listening

Among the many communication strategies at your disposal, active listening is arguably the most effective, especially when relating to a loved one with mental illness. It's more than just hearing the words that are spoken; it's about understanding the complete message being sent, both verbally and nonverbally.

Active listening involves fully focusing on the speaker, not interrupting, and responding thoughtfully rather than reactively. This mindful approach to communication allows you to embrace empathy and validation, opening a genuine connection and understanding between yourself and your loved one.

To manage effectively, it helps to be aware of the physical cues that may reveal what's going on beneath the surface. This includes observing body language, facial expressions, and tone of voice, which often convey more truth than spoken words themselves. By paying attention to these subtle signs, you can better understand your loved one's needs and emotional state, fostering an environment of compassion and trust.

When you engage in active listening, you avoid "cross-talk," or conversations where each participant is merely waiting for their turn to speak. It's beneficial to ensure you provide a safe space where your loved one feels seen, heard, and not judged. This is achieved by expressing your understanding of what they're sharing, even if you don't entirely relate or agree. It's not about having all the answers; it's about showing a genuine desire to comprehend their perspective.

It's essential to remember that active listening doesn't mean you're relinquishing your opportunity to share your feelings or feedback. However, it's crucial to do so in a considerate way that respects the speaker's experience and feelings. Ask for permission to share your thoughts and ensure the timing is right. The goal is to foster emotional safety to encourage open and honest communication.

One practical active listening technique is paraphrasing. This is when you repeat in your own words what you understood the speaker to say. This shows the speaker that you're engaged and trying to comprehend their point of view. Furthermore, it offers an opportunity for clarification if you misunderstood anything.

Another beneficial approach is using open-ended questions. These are inquiries that can't be answered with a simple yes or no. They encourage the speaker to share more in-depth insights, thoughts, and feelings, promoting a deeper understanding and connection between the two parties involved.

Validating feelings is yet another powerful aspect of active listening. By acknowledging the emotional experience of the person talking—without trying to change it, fix it, or offer unsolicited advice—you communicate your acceptance and understanding. Remember, validation doesn't mean agreement; it's just an acknowledgment of the person's experience.

Part of active listening is about displaying patience. Understand that expressing feelings or thoughts, especially around mental health, can be challenging and intimidating. Allow your loved one to take their time, and avoid rushing them or making assumptions about what they're trying to convey.

Keep in mind that active listening is a skill, and like any skill, it can be improved with practice. Challenge yourself to employ these techniques in your everyday conversations. The more you practice, the more they'll become an integral part of your communication arsenal, thus enhancing your ability to support your loved one.

Active listening as part of effective communication strategies is all about building a bridge of empathy, respect, and understanding. It's not about making judgments or asserting your point of view. Instead, it's about being fully present and in the moment, embracing the messages spoken to you and the unsaid ones hanging in the silent spaces.

There will be times when active listening will be challenging, emotionally draining even, especially when the conversation touches raw nerves. On these occasions, remind yourself that it's perfectly okay to take a step back and take a deep breath. It's important when having difficult conversations to know when to take a break. After all, preserving your emotional well-being is just as essential as comprehending your loved one's inner world. However, as important as it is to take a break during tough conversations, it is equally important to come back to the conversation in a timely manner in order to get the issue at hand resolved so there isn't any negativity lingering over the relationship with your loved one.

Finally, it's crucial to remember that as beneficial as active listening is, it's not a cure or a fix for mental health issues. It's a tool, a powerful one, to build understanding, trust, and mutual respect. At the end of the day, supporting a loved one with a mental illness necessitates a multifaceted approach, and active listening is one integral part of this approach.

Practicing active listening can be enlightening and deeply rewarding. It can foster profound connections, nurture trust, and inspire healing, acceptance, and growth in your relationships-especially with your loved one living with mental illness. All it requires is a little patience, effort, and an open heart.

Non-Verbal Communication

As you continue the journey to assist loved ones through mental illness, your ability to communicate effectively becomes vital. A crucial part of this communication process, which is often understated, is the use of non-verbal cues.

Non-verbal communication refers to the transmission of messages or signals through a nonverbal platform such as eye contact, facial expressions, gestures, posture, and the distance between two individuals. These silent conversations can speak volumes about a person's feelings, attitudes, and intentions.

However, when someone is suffering from a mental illness, their non-verbal communication may be altered or misunderstood. Thus, interpreting these signals correctly can help you better understand and connect with your loved one.

For example, consider the role of body language in non-verbal communication. A slouched posture or crossed arms might indicate feelings of sadness or discomfort, signaling to you their mental state without the need for words. Similarly, their tone of voice, volume, rate of speech, and vocal quality play significant roles as well. A timid tone might indicate nervousness, while fast pacing could signify worry or stress.

While these signals are crucial, interpreting them accurately can be challenging. We often misunderstand or overlook these cues. For instance, your loved one might repeatedly rub their hands, signaling anxiety or stress, but it's easy to miss this gesture if you're not intentionally looking for it and understanding its meaning.

Facial expressions are another significant aspect of non-verbal communication. They can convey a wealth of emotions—from happiness and surprise to anger, sadness, and fear. Consider how much you can glean from a loved one's face alone, even with limited verbal interaction. However, understand that interpretations may vary across different cultures. For instance, direct eye contact might signify attentiveness in one culture and disrespect in another.

Acknowledge the language of the eyes, as the eyes often betray what words conceal. Prolonged eye contact can suggest interest, respect, or attraction, but in other contexts, it could be a sign of aggression. Stillness or lack of blinking suggests deep concentration or engagement, while frequent blinking may indicate distress or discomfort.

Physical touch presents another layer of complexity to non-verbal communication. While a comforting hug can be reassuring, if done without considering the receiver's comfort level, it can lead to discomfort and a sense of violation. With your loved ones battling mental illness, it's essential to consider their personal space boundaries.

The concept of personal space, or proximity, differs from person to person. Often, when a person is comfortable around you, they tend to reduce the personal space between the two of you. However, while dealing with mental health issues, a person may require a larger personal space. Acknowledging and honoring this space can make them more comfortable and open.

Also, the environment itself communicates a non-verbal message. For example, engaging your loved one in a quiet, calm, well-lit room might make them feel safe and open to conversation than a loud, crowded, chaotic setting.

Learning to interpret non-verbal cues accurately requires keen observation, patience, and practice. It's like tuning into a silent frequency that communicates the unsaid and unseen. Understanding this language can greatly enhance your interactions with your loved one and foster a mutual understanding.

Consider your loved one's unique personality and behavior when interpreting their nonverbal cues. Be open-minded and avoid making hasty judgments based on biased perceptions or previous experiences. This requires patience, understanding, and empathy. Remember, the aim is not to judge but to better understand.

In conclusion, non-verbal communication is a powerful tool for connecting with a loved one suffering from mental illness. When combined with active listening and understanding, it serves as a beacon, guiding your loved one through their often daunting mental landscape. It illuminates their truth, helping you bridge the gap between what is spoken and what is felt.

Chapter 3 Key Take Aways

1. It isn't just about what you say, but how you say it, how well you listen, and the non-verbal cues you convey.

2. You want your loved one to feel heard, valued, and understood. You're not just waiting to speak; you're hearing, absorbing, and responding to the emotions behind the words.

3. It's important to discover and understand the physical, psychological, and social barriers.

Chapter 4:
Helping a Loved One with Mental Illness

Having brushed up on our communication skills, we now wade into the heart of our journey together-the practical and emotional elements of helping a loved one manage mental illness. As a caregiver, you shoulder immense responsibility in assisting with tasks such as ensuring medication compliance and helping with job acquisition and retention. However, this role isn't solely defined by functional support. It also encompasses providing emotional bolstering, becoming a reliable source of solace and validation in the often isolating domain of mental illness. This dichotomy, of hands-on assistance and emotional sustenance, is a balancing act, one that requires patience and resilience. It's important to remember though, that even amidst this flurry of responsibility, you can't pour from an empty cup. To be an effective caregiver, you need to make sure you're taking care of your own wellbeing.

The Role of the Caregiver

Helping a loved one navigate through the rough waves of a mental illness can be as challenging as it is rewarding. As a caregiver, you play a critical role in your loved one's journey towards betterment. That role can include several facets-from emotional support and physical assistance to aiding them with their critical assignments.

The role of a caregiver in mental health can often feel like a balancing act. As a caregiver, you want to provide support while respecting your loved ones' autonomy and encouraging them to take an active role in their recovery. This requires a delicate blend of empathy, understanding, and resilience.

One of the most essential roles you can serve as a caregiver is that of an ally. Mental illness can often set us apart from others, leading to feelings of isolation and despair. Your loved one needs an advocate, a person who stands by their side in spite of their mental health condition, who believes in their ability to recover, and who can shine a light on their worth when they're unable to see it themselves.

Another core facet of your role as a caregiver is education. Educate yourself about mental illness. This knowledge is a powerful tool that can prove invaluable in combatting the stigma of mental illness, understanding its implications, and knowing the best way to manage it. This education doesn't only mean understanding the specific diagnosis, but also being familiar with the signs of potential crisis, possible side-effects of medications, and the strategies for effective communication.

Being emotionally available for your loved one is another big part of your role, albeit a challenging one. It's about being a patient listener, understanding and validating their feelings, comforting them during tough times, and celebrating their small wins. Your loved one might not always be able to articulate what they're feeling or going through, and that's where your understanding and validation is needed.

Serving as an advocate for their healthcare is yet another aspect of your caregiver role. This could involve accompanying them to physical and mental health appointments, ensuring clear communication between them and their health care providers, and monitoring their medication intake. Remember, you play an important part in their treatment plan, since you're often the one on ground zero observing and reporting symptoms and changes.

Helping them maintain their daily routine and independence as much as possible is crucial. This includes supporting them in their hygiene, nutrition, and bringing continuity in their sleep patterns, etc. Consider using gentle prompts, reminders, and encouragement without commandeering their lives.

The multimodal role of a caregiver can sometimes feel burdensome. It's important to remember to take care of you too. Neglecting your physical and mental health can result in burnout, which isn't beneficial for either of you.

Being a mental health caregiver also involves managing logistics. This includes support with transportation for appointments, administrative help with filing insurance claims, and managing finances. The logistical side of caregiving can be tedious, but it's crucial for efficient and smooth progress.

As a caregiver, you need to be adaptable and flexible. Mental illnesses can often be unpredictable, symptoms might change, treatment methods could be altered. Your loved one might have good days and very hard days. Adaptability and patience becomes your superpower.

You also have the role of bringing normalcy into their lives. Engaging them in everyday activities, fostering social interactions and ensuring their inclusion in family activities can significantly contribute to their mental well-being.

Your role extends to being a provider of peace and calm in your loved one's world. Ensuring your loved one's environment is safe, free from unnecessary stress, and conducive to their recovery, is an aspect you could oversee.

One of the hardest, yet most rewarding aspects of being a caregiver is being someone who instills hope. Dealing with a mental illness can often seem overwhelming and endless. Your relentless optimism and unwavering faith in their recovery can serve as a beacon of hope in their darkest times.

The role of a caregiver isn't straightforward, it isn't easy, but it's incredibly important. It requires perseverance, patience and a whole lot of love. Remember, just as they are on a journey, so are you.

Assistive Tasks for the Caregiver

As a caregiver for a loved one with a mental illness, you'll encounter a wide range of responsibilities. These tasks often include providing physical, emotional, and social support, aiding with treatment compliance, and ensuring a structured, low-stress environment. We'll delve into the specifics of these roles throughout this section.

Perhaps one of the most crucial roles as a caregiver is helping the individual adhere to their prescribed treatment plan. The benefits of medications are unmistakable, yet the rate of non-adherence is high. It is crucial to communicate openly and honestly with your loved one about the importance of their medication routine. You might play an active role in reminding them to take medication, pick up prescriptions, and check-in with their healthcare provider regularly whether in person or via telemedicine.

You can help by setting reminders or alarms for medications, packaging the medication in easily accessible pill boxes, and maintaining an accurate record of medicines taken. It's essential, however, not to push or apply too much pressure as this could lead to resistance and further complicate the situation. A gentle, supportive approach tends to work best.

Regular appointments with mental health professionals are essential to ensure the ongoing efficacy of treatment, keep track of progress, and address any arising concerns promptly. As a caregiver, you can assist your loved one in scheduling and remembering these appointments. Perhaps even attend some of these appointments together if your loved one is comfortable with it. This can provide you with better understanding about what they are going through and how you can assist in their recovery process.

Joining the workforce is another critical step towards recovery for many people with mental illnesses. However, initiating and maintaining employment can present significant challenges. As a caregiver, you can aid your loved one in this transition, whether it's providing assistance with job applications, providing transportation to interviews, or offering emotional support through the inevitable ups and downs.

By promoting a routine, you can help your loved one manage their stress levels and foster a sense of accomplishment. It's equally important to celebrate their work accomplishments, no matter how small they seem. Commend them for taking baby steps and remind them that personal growth isn't measurable by size but by progress.

Physical assistance also falls under the umbrella of caregiving. This can range from helping with everyday tasks such as meal preparation, cleaning, or shopping to more involved tasks like ensuring safe usage of potentially dangerous household items. Remember, each individual's need for physical assistance will differ based on their specific set of symptoms and the severity of their illness.

Emotional support might just be the most critical element in the journey of mental health recovery. Be there for your loved one. Make sure they know that they're not alone, that their experiences and feelings are valid. Encourage them to express their thoughts and feelings and show them that it's okay not to be okay.

Provide consistent positivity and reassurance that things will get better. Actively seek out small joyous moments or amusing activities to do together. The path to recovery is often more bearable when they perceive love, patience, and genuine care from those around them.

However, your role as a caregiver goes beyond merely assisting in the practicalities of daily life. It's also about being a steady source of unwavering support and love. Ensure that they never feel like a burden, but rather, let them know they're valued, loved, and that their mental illness doesn't define them.

Support their interests and passions, encourage them to pursue hobbies and distractions that bring them pleasure. This can be beneficial not only for their mental health but also for their overall wellness. Additionally, this could help them rebuild self-confidence and find a sense of purpose.

Don't hesitate to seek help. If the journey becomes too overwhelming, there are resources available specifically for caregivers. Support groups, therapy sessions, helplines, and informational resources can aid you in your challenging yet much-needed role. Remember, caregiving isn't about being perfect. It's about being there, doing your best, and showing your love in every action.

Being a mental health caregiver might not be a task you'd ever anticipated, but with every challenge comes growth. By opening up your heart and extending your strength to someone else, you're helping guide them on their journey to recovery, and this is a truly life-affirming privilege that builds resilience in both of you.

Helping them to take their mental health medication as prescribed

When a loved one is living with a mental health disorder, ensuring they take their prescribed medications becomes a significant responsibility. Adherence to medication not only helps manage symptoms, but also plays a pivotal role in their health and well-being.

Beginning on this journey may be challenging. Disorientation, mistrust, and miscommunication can become stumbling blocks. However, with patience, persistence, and a desire to understand, you can truly support your loved one in their medication regimen.

The first step toward understanding involves educating yourself about the prescribed medications. Understand their benefits, side effects, and potential risks. Ask the health professional questions, clarify doubts, and ensure you have the informational groundwork to guide your loved one effectively. Remember, knowledge empowers, and in this context, provides the backbone for guided support.

Establishing a routine is key. Most psychiatric medications require regular intake, often at the same time each day. A routine aids compliance by merging medication intake within the rhythm of life. Use tools such as medication organizers, mobile applications, or even simple reminders in places where your loved one spends time.

However, remember that routines should not feel rigid. Instead, they should complement and adjust to the ebb and flow of your loved one's life. Promoting autonomy in this process can aid adherence to the medication routine and cultivate a sense of self-agency in your loved one.

Impersonality can inhibit this process. Therefore, a crucial part of this journey is embracing empathy. Realize that your loved one is not their illness; they are individuals living with a condition. This can cause fear, anxiety, and frustration. Being empathetic to these experiences can connect you with them on a deeper level, making the process smoother and more effective.

Encourage open discussions around the medications. A space where your loved one feels understood and can air their concerns, doubts or fears can facilitate better adherence to medications. Remember, silencing fears only gives the fears power. In responding with compassion and validation, you can help alleviate any anxiety related to medication.

Engage your loved one in creating a contingency plan to manage missed doses or other medication-related problems. Make sure this plan accounts for their needs, respects their autonomy, and offers realistic solutions. This proactive approach can create a sense of security around the medication regimen, and further supports adherence to treatment.

Monitor the effects of the medication. This can involve observing mood shifts, physical changes, or any behavioral differences. Though it's important not to assume every change is due to medication, they could simply be having a bad day, like everyone has from time to time. Keeping records and notes can help in discussions with the medical professional and provide important feedback on optimization of treatment.

Provide praise and positive feedback when your loved one adheres to their medication regimen. Reinforcement through regular recognition of their efforts can foster feelings of achievement and motivate continued compliance. Small rewards can go a long way in encouraging a positive attitude towards medication adherence.

Despite all our efforts, there may be times when your loved one refuses to take their medication. It's essential, albeit challenging, to handle these moments with patience and understanding. Empathize with their feelings, explore their reasons, and suggest alternative ways to approach the situation.

Above all else, remember that care must be reciprocal. Helping a loved one manage their medication involves your well-being as well. Prioritize self-care, ensuring that you are both mentally and physically capable of extending support. It's OK to seek your own support system, to ask for help when needed, or to simply take a break and recharge.

Supporting a loved one with their medication is a significant task, one that can often seem daunting. Along the journey, there may be doubts, frustration, and a feeling of being overwhelmed. However, embedded in these challenges are moments of profound connection, genuine kindness, and the fortitude of the human spirit.

Remember, you're not alone in this journey, even if it sometimes feels like an uphill climb. You're forming the cornerstone of your loved one's support system. Your patience, understanding, empathy, and love can play a crucial role in their mental health recovery.

Assist, guide, and support, but also empower. Encourage your loved one to take an active role in caring for their mental health. By doing so, you are not just helping them stabilize and thrive amidst their condition, you're also empowering them with a newfound sense of self and autonomy. An autonomy where medication becomes an ally, rather than an adversary, in their journey towards mental health.

Helping them to make and keep appointments

Ensuring that your loved one consistently attends medical and therapeutic appointments is a crucial aspect of helping them manage their mental illness. It's more than simply setting a reminder or driving them to the clinic. It involves understanding their resistance, offering support, and encouraging self-reliance.

Often, individuals struggling with mental illness might find the task of scheduling or keeping appointments overwhelming. This may stem from a sense of fear or anxiety surrounding their condition and the treatment process. In such cases, your role as a caregiver would involve addressing these fears and providing reassurance. Walk them through the process, explaining its importance and how it will aid their recovery.

Moreover, foster an environment of open communication. Encourage them to share their thoughts about the upcoming appointments, whether they have fears, concerns, or questions. By acknowledging and normalizing their feelings, you not only reassure them but also build trust and strengthen your relationship.

Once you've addressed their reservations and they agree to set an appointment, assist in the task. Let them take the lead, but be available for support. This can involve helping to find a mental health professional, offering to make the call, or sitting with them during the process. Depending on their comfort level and current mental state, they may want to do that on their own or appreciate your assistance.

Remember, keeping the appointments is just as crucial as making them. As a caregiver, it's important to create a system that will help them remember these appointments. This could be setting reminders on their phone, creating an easily-visible schedule on a whiteboard, or setting up a shared calendar. Explore different options and find what works best for them.

While reminders are beneficial, the goal should be teaching and encouraging your loved one to take responsibility for their healthcare schedule. You can incorporate this into your daily interactions, emphasizing the value of structure and time management in recovery. Acknowledging their steps towards self-management can be a great confidence boost and further motivate them.

Consistency is key in outpatient mental health treatment and the continuous cycle of scheduling, keeping, and reflecting on appointments creates a necessary structure that aids in recovery. Encourage them to reflect on what was discussed during their sessions and how they can implement the learned coping strategies and behaviors into their everyday life. Similar to building any habit, turning treatment participation into a routine can help tremendously.

At times, despite best efforts, your loved one may refuse to attend appointments. It's vital to approach these situations with compassion. Instead of expressing anger or disappointment, ask them about their reasoning and listen to their concerns. Engage in supportive decision-making dialogue, reiterating how beneficial these appointments are for their well-being.

In circumstances when the individual repeatedly misses appointments, it may be worth exploring alternatives. If physical attendance is the issue, consider remote therapy options–a growing area in mental health care. Online therapy can be a lower-stress alternative, eliminating travel and waiting in unfamiliar surroundings.

Helping a loved one with mental illness to make and keep appointments might be challenging and require patience. Yet, in the long run, it helps them establish an indispensable routine, develop self-dependency, and move towards improved mental health. Your role as a caregiver is to support and guide them towards these steps of self-care. Your encouragement can be instrumental in the progress they make.

Beyond schedules and reminders, remember to check in on how your loved one feels about their ongoing treatment. Give them space and opportunity to voice any concerns, and affirm their experiences. Mental health treatment can be a long, winding journey, and feeling heard can make a world of difference for someone navigating it.

Understand that there are good days and bad days. There will be appointments that go great, returning with newfound insights, and some that could be disheartening. As a caregiver, be there for them in both instances. Celebrate their small victories, and provide comfort during the inevitable challenges. It's this consistent, loving support that makes a sustainable difference.

At the end of the day, helping them make and keep appointments is about more than providing a ride or setting reminders. It's about fostering self-management, reminding them that they're not alone, and walking alongside them on their path of recovery. Your role as caregiver plays an integral part; your support and involvement can aid their personal growth, help to maintain their routine, and, ultimately, contribute to the improvement of their mental health.

Helping them to get and keep a job

One of the crucial steps towards recovery and normalcy for a person with mental illness is finding a job and maintaining it. Not only does it boost their self-esteem, but it also creates a sense of purpose and structure that significantly aids in mental wellness.

It's essential to understand that as a caregiver, your role is to support and not push your loved one into a job blindly. The transition back into the working world can be taxing and stressful for individuals grappling with mental health issues. Therefore, your loved one must understand the significance of a job and be willing to take up the responsibility.

Having conversations about employment can feel overwhelming. Frame the discussion in a way that emphasises the positive aspects of working, such as feeling productive, social interaction, and financial independence. It's also beneficial to discuss the possible challenges that might present themselves, to prepare your loved one on handling them.

Leverage resources available like vocational rehabilitation counselors or mental health professionals who are trained to help mentally ill individuals prepare for, find, and maintain employment. They can provide valuable skill training, resume writing aid, and advice on the interview process.

When starting the job hunt, focus on searching for jobs that match your loved one's skills and comfort level. Maybe they're more comfortable with part-time work to start, or perhaps remote work could be a better alternative given their current state. The employment environment plays a significant role in their overall mental wellbeing, so ensuring they're comfortable is paramount.

Help your loved one draft their resume, emphasizing their abilities and achievements instead of a chronological job history that might be spotty due to their illness. Encourage your loved one to focus on positions suitable for their strengths, as it will boost their confidence and reduce job-related stress.

Keep in mind that interviewing for jobs can cause anxiety and panic in someone dealing with a mental illness. Practice mock interviews with them, noting their body language, maintaining eye contact, addressing their potential employer confidently, and answering questions honestly but tactfully.

Remember that your loved one has a legal right to keep their mental illness private from potential employers unless they choose to disclose it. The decision to be open about their mental illness at work is intensely personal and subjective. Again, guide them through this thought process, weighing the pros and cons carefully.

Furthermore, remember that sometimes it is hard to take advice or constructive criticism from people who we are close with, like friends and family; so remember your loved one might not prefer to have you specifically help with resume writing and mock interviews. For situations such as this, there are programs that offer what's called a job coach for people with a diagnosed mental illness. Instead of physically helping them with all the hands on tasks of finding and landing a job, you can help them get connected with a job coach in their area.

Once they land a job, the real work begins. Their new job will present a set of challenges, such as managing stress levels, maintaining performance, dealing with social interactions, and possibly handling stigma. As a caregiver, highlighting coping mechanisms like time management, creating a routine, or reaching out when they need help can be incredibly beneficial.

Encourage your loved one to set achievable goals and milestones, focus on what they can control, and not be too hard on themselves if they stumble. Remind them about the importance of self-care, taking time to de-stress, and ensuring they maintain a balance between work and leisure.

Having regular check-ins with your loved one can help to understand their work situation better. Have discussions about their job satisfaction, any struggles they're facing, their coping mechanisms, and whether they're managing their work-life balance. Such conversations can give you insights into their mental wellness regarding their work environment.

Keep in mind that it's okay if things don't work out at first. It might take a few tries, but each failure is a step closer to finding a job that will work for them. As a caregiver, maintaining positivity and offering continual encouragement in such situations is necessary. Sometimes simply just being there as a person they can vent to about work-related stressors is the best way you can support them in the realm of employment search and continued employment.

Helping your loved one to get and keep a job is not a straightforward process. It's about maintaining patience, showing understanding, and helping them navigate through this complex journey towards betterment. Remember, your unending support and faith in their capabilities can greatly affect their motivation levels and overall growth.

Last but certainly not least, don't lose sight of your well-being in this process. It can be taxing for caregivers to navigate this journey. Ensure you take time out for self-care and seek help and support when needed. Caring for yourself is as essential as caring for your loved one.

Physical Assistance

When it comes to caring for a loved one with mental illness, providing physical assistance can sometimes be as crucial as offering emotional support. Several aspects, ranging from helping manage their medication and health appointments to aiding in their daily activities, fall under this domain. Let's delve deeper into each of these components.

Handling medication is a major part of physical support. You might need to remind your loved one to take their prescribed medicines, which can be challenging if memory issues or reluctance are part of their mental illness. Educating yourself about their medication-its administration, possible side effects, and interactions-can also help you interact more efficiently with their healthcare providers.

Next comes the responsibility of making and managing your loved one's healthcare appointments. People living with mental illness often struggle with organizing and tracking important dates, including their doctor and therapy sessions. By taking an active role in scheduling these and offering to accompany them, you can ensure they are receiving the necessary professional help.

Another significant aspect of physical assistance involves facilitating and maintaining their personal hygiene and cleanliness. This can involve a wide spectrum of tasks, depending on their functional capacity. It might range from gentle prompts to brush their teeth, to more direct help like assisting them in the shower. Respect their autonomy as much as possible while ensuring they are keeping up with these necessary daily routines.

Mental illness can sometimes make the basic act of feeding oneself a challenge. Helping your loved one maintain a balanced diet can significantly contribute to their overall well-being. Coordinate meal planning and preparation, help with shopping for nutritious foods within their budget, or set alarms and reminders to eat. Remember that good nutrition can contribute to the effectiveness of their treatment. Vitamins that are important for improved mental health are vitamins B, D, C, magnesium, zinc, omega 3 fatty acids, and probiotics. Make sure your loved one is taking a daily multivitamin and eating foods rich in these mental health vitamins. Vitamin B rich foods include eggs, liver, shellfish, crab, fermented cheese, tofu, salmon, leafy greens, oysters, chicken, legumes, turkey, and yogurt. Vitamin D rich foods include salmon, sardines, tuna, egg yolks, and fortified dairy. Vitamin C rich foods include citrus fruits, peppers, strawberries, and broccoli. Magnesium rich foods include seeds, almonds, spinach, cashews, and peanuts. Zinc rich foods include lamb, pumpkin seeds, garbanzo beans, cashews, yogurt, mushrooms, and spinach. And omega 3 fatty acid rich foods include fish, chia seeds, walnuts, seaweed, seeds, and olive oil.

Exercise promotes overall health and is known to boost mood, making it beneficial for those with mental illness. You can lend physical support by creating and maintaining an exercise routine suitable for your loved one's capabilities, encouraging them to engage in it regularly. This might involve anything from a simple walk around the block to structured workouts or games.

You can also assist in the overall maintenance of their living environment. Ensure their home is not only clean but also safe, quiet, tranquil, and suitable for recovery. This might mean doing household chores or making sure the house is well-stocked with all the amenities they need.

Sleep often becomes elusive and disturbed for those dealing with mental illnesses. Ensuring that they have a comfortable, quiet, and dark environment to sleep in can do wonders for their health. Their room should be a space of calm and tranquility, comforting and conducive to relaxation. If your loved one struggles with sleep things you could suggest they try is spraying lavender on their pillow, taking a warm bath or shower before bed, drinking a warm glass of milk before bed, sticking to a bedtime routine, sleeping with a weighted blanket, mindfulness meditation, having a white noise machine next to their bed or there are some videos on the internet that play calming noises with dark-colored screens to help with sleep.

As a caregiver, aiding them to maintain a structured daily routine could be another vital part of your role. Individuals with mental illness might struggle with time management and organization, making their days seem chaotic and overwhelming. Reminding them about important tasks or helping them follow a schedule can bring stability and predictability, mitigating anxiety.

If your loved one is employed or seeking employment, providing support in this area is essential too. This might involve driving them to and from work, helping manage work-related stress, or even assisting them in searching for a job that suits their abilities and current mental wellness state.

In instances where your loved one's mental illness significantly impairs their mobility, your role might include physical tasks such as moving them in and out of bed, aiding them in walking, or even taking them on wheelchair-accessible outings. These tasks, although often physically demanding for you as a caregiver, can greatly enhance their quality of life.

In the realm of physical assistance, one must never overlook the importance of touch. Simple acts like holding their hand, giving a reassuring hug, or a pat on the back can communicate love, warmth, and reassurance effectively. Remember to always respect their comfort zone and personal boundaries when offering such physical consolation.

Mental illness can make individuals feel disconnected from the world around them. By providing transportation for outings to the park or visits to friends and family, you can help keep them socially connected and involved in activities that they enjoy, aiding in their recovery.

It's important to note that providing physical assistance does not mean doing everything for your loved one or taking complete control. Make sure to respect their autonomy and encourage them to do things for themselves as much as they can. Your aim should be to empower them, not make them feel helpless or incapacitated.

All in all, providing physical assistance for a loved one with mental illness encompasses a wide range of responsibilities and tasks, each as crucial as the next. Remember that while this journey can be challenging, by demonstrating patience, compassion, and understanding, you're making a significant impact on your loved one's life and recovery journey.

Emotional Support

When a loved one is living with a mental illness, offering emotional support may often be one of the greatest challenges, yet it's also one of the most crucial facets in their journey towards recovery or management of the illness. This path will be fraught with emotional turmoil, not just for your loved one, but for you as a caregiver too. Acknowledging this emotional journey is the first step towards providing effective emotional support.

One of the most crucial aspects of emotional support is patience. Mental illness is not something that can be overcome overnight. It requires time, effort, and, most importantly, a lot of patience. Reinforce to your loved one that it's okay to take time to heal, that there's no rush, and they don't have to put unnecessary pressure on themselves.

In addition to patience, the emotional support toolbox should also include empathy. Empathy allows you to put yourself in their shoes and understand what they're going through. This understanding can give you insights into their experiences and emotions, which in return will help you offer comfort, encouragement, and support in a way that truly resonates with them. It is not always about understanding their emotions, but most importantly, validating them.

Importantly, it's also helpful to learn to be comfortable with silence. Sometimes, a loved one with mental illness may not want to talk about their feelings or experiences, or may find it too difficult to put them into words. Carving out space for silence signals to them that you're there to support them without any demand to communicate if they're not ready.

To provide emotional support, being non-judgmental is paramount. Let your loved one reminisce or express feelings without fearing criticism or judgement. They are likely already dealing with a lot internally, and the last thing they may need is condemnation or criticism.

Cultivating an open dialogue about emotions and mental health is another key strategy. Eliminate the taboo of mental health and make it a topic that can be openly discussed. Encourage your loved one to share their feelings and offer reassurance that it's okay to have these conversations.

Let them define their own experiences. As a caregiver, it's easy to think you understand someone's experiences or feelings better than they do. However, their emotional experience is uniquely their own. Let them define what they're going through, and how they want to deal with it. This personal empowerment is an important part of their healing process.

Keeping your own emotions in check is a vital part of offering emotional support. It's normal to feel frustrated, agitated, or sad when a loved one is struggling. However, expressing these emotions can affect the emotional harmony of the individual dealing with mental health issues. Thus, finding ways to manage your emotions is crucial.

A soft, positive approach is another way of providing emotional support. Instead of making promises that things will improve immediately, assure them that they're not alone in their struggle, and that you're there to help them through it. Express positive thoughts about their strength and resilience, and remind them of their progress, however small it may seem.

Acknowledge their struggles and pain without trying to fix them instantaneously. As a caregiver, it's instinctive to want to fix problems and make things better. But in this case, offering emotional support often means simply acknowledging their pain and reaffirming that it's okay to be having a hard time. Expressing empathy for what they're experiencing is a powerful form of support.

Being present physically is not enough. True emotional support lies in being mentally and emotionally present. Whether it's through sharing a quiet moment, listening actively, or validating their feelings, ensure that your loved one knows you're psychologically present for them.

Avoid stigmatizing language or behavior. Stigma can create an environment of shame, fear, and silence, severely hindering the healing process. Affirm to your loved one that mental illness doesn't define their worth or value, and never label them by their illness.

Empower them to make decisions about their own mental health. While it's tempting to take control and make decisions for them, empowering your loved one to take charge and express what they need can be tremendously beneficial for their recovery and self-esteem.

Finally, suggest therapy and counseling when appropriate and ensure to present it as a positive and potentially beneficial thing. If they're ready to consider it, help them explore this option by providing needed information or accompanying them for sessions, if they are comfortable with it.

Remember, your emotional support can be a lifeline, providing your loved one with the assurance that they're not alone in their journey. However, while supporting them, don't neglect your own needs and emotions. Balancing your well-being with providing emotional support to your loved one will make the journey smoother for both of you.

Mental Illness And Addiction

Often times people with mental illness also struggle with addictions such as drugs and alcohol, gambling, sex/pornography, shopping, etc. There are several reasons why this may occur. **Mental illness can contribute to addiction.** Poor impulse control is a symptom of many mental illnesses, which can hinder one's ability to say no to certain substances or behaviors. Poor impulse control, sensation-seeking, feelings of invincibility, and being prone to higher levels of boredom are all due to a disruption in levels of key proteins involved in neurotransmission in the brain's reward pathway. People with mental illness often turn to drugs and alcohol, gambling, sex, and shopping to get the adrenaline rush in order to substitute for the lack of dopamine being produced in the brain. These behaviors may temporarily relieve some symptoms of mental illness, however, they can make the symptoms worse over time. Additionally, brain changes in people with mental illness may enhance the rewarding effects of these behaviors, making it more likely they will continue with the behavior while also increasing the amount and duration of the behavior or substance. **Common risk factors can contribute to both mental illness and addictive behaviors.** Mental illness and addiction can run in families, meaning certain genes may be a risk factor. Environmental factors, such as trauma, can cause genetic changes in the brain causing mental illness and/or addictive behaviors. **Substance use can contribute to mental illness.** Substance use can trigger changes in brain structure that can make a person more likely to develop a mental illness.

There is very little to be done to prevent addiction in persons with mental illness aside from their lack of desire for addictive behaviors and their ability to stick with their mental health treatment plan. Therefore, you can help prevent them from experiencing addictive behaviors and substances by being a positive influence in their life and encouraging them to follow their mental health treatment plan.

If your loved one does become addicted to an unhealthy activity or substance it is important that they have an integrated approach to treatment where they can work on both their mental health and addiction at the same time. This integrated approach may include individual therapy, group therapy, medication, behavioral therapy, assistance with detoxification, assistance with managing withdrawal symptoms, and lifestyle changes that may include moving to a new community, ending friendships/relationships and starting new ones; staying away from certain neighborhoods, stores, medications/substances, and events.

Your role in caring for your loved one with mental illness and addiction issues is to ensure they are meeting with their mental health care and addiction team and following their treatment plan. Following their treatment plan includes the above mentioned lifestyle changes. As their caregiver, you can help them to make positive choices in these lifestyle changes, such as ensuring they delete certain phone numbers of people who aid in their addiction, ensuring they get on the banned list for casinos and other locations that contribute to their addiction, go with them to support group meetings, keep them occupied and make plans with them that does not include locations and activities where they would typically perform their addictive behavior, and finally, you can simply be there to talk to them when they are getting the urge to perform their addictive behavior of choice.

<u>Chapter 4 Key Take Aways</u>

1. You should aim to provide support while respecting your loved one's autonomy and encouraging them to take an active role in their recovery.

2. Key facets of a caregiver is to be an ally, to be an advocate, to educate yourself about mental illness, and providing emotional and physical support.

3. Make sure you practice self-care. Do not neglect your own needs.

Chapter 5:
Building a Positive Relationship

To foster a positive relationship with a loved one suffering from mental illness, begin with setting healthy boundaries. These boundaries are critical in maintaining a balance between caring for your loved one and your personal needs. Ensuring personal space and personal time is respected can uphold the mental wellbeing of both parties. Develop an understanding of their needs; comprehend their experiences, struggles, and emotions. This asks for empathy: envision being in their shoes but remember to separate their feelings from yours. It allows for more concrete support when both emotional and psychological boundaries are clear. Equally important in cultivating a successful relationship is fostering mutual respect and trust. Involve them in shared decision making, communicate honestly, show devout care, and respect their individuality. Remember, maintaining trust is a continual process and should be preserved even during strained periods. Building a positive relationship with a mentally ill loved one demands patience but is instrumental in creating an environment conducive to recovery and healing.

Setting Healthy Boundaries

One of the most crucial aspects of building a positive relationship with a loved one who has a mental illness is the establishment of healthy boundaries. Boundaries are essentially guidelines or rules determined by an individual for their self-protection. They portray the emotional, mental, and physical limits an individual has established to identify reasonable and permissible ways they can be treated by others.

It's essential for caregivers to understand that setting boundaries is not an act of selfishness; rather, it's an act of self-care. Think of it as outlining a safety zone around yourself, not to isolate you from your loved one, but to protect your wellbeing while providing them with the best possible care and support.

The need for boundaries often stems from a place of love and compassion, both for your loved one and yourself. Although it might feel uncomfortable initially, it's necessary for preserving your emotional, physical, and mental health. Just as a doctor would use gloves and sanitizers to protect themselves in a medical procedure, boundaries act as emotional tools of safeguarding for caregivers.

Healthy boundaries can also help manage expectations and reduce potential disagreements or misunderstandings. Specifically, when you communicate your limits to your loved one, it provides them with a clear understanding of what they can expect from you.

It's important to remember that boundaries are unique to each person and relationship. What feels burdensome or overwhelming to one caregiver, another might handle comfortably. The key is to understand and respect your own limits. Don't measure your boundaries against those of anyone else; your journey is unique and so are your needs.

Recognizing the need for boundaries is one part of the equation, but the real challenge lies in the act of setting and maintaining them. In fact, it's common to experience feelings of guilt during this process, but remind yourself that this is a necessary step towards achieving a balanced caregiving relationship.

The development of healthy boundaries begins with self-awareness, in recognizing when you're feeling deprived, frustrated, exhausted, or resentful. These emotions often signal that your needs aren't being met and boundaries are being crossed. Explore these feelings, identify your needs, and assert them with clear, straightforward communication.

Remember to convey your boundaries in a respectful yet firm manner without letting guilt or fear hold you back. Be specific in your conversation; clearly state what you're comfortable with, and articulate the actions or behaviors you find unacceptable. It's also essential to make sure your body language aligns with your words, reflecting your determination and commitment.

It's important to note that setting boundaries isn't a one-time event, but a continuous process. Flexibility is crucial, as you might need to revisit and adjust your boundaries based on changes in your loved one's condition or your own personal circumstances.

Invite your loved one to respect your boundaries. It can take time for them to adjust to new guidelines, so patience is key. Understand that they may not always agree with your limits, and that's alright. It can be a challenging transition, and it might take some time for them to fully understand and respect these measures. It may also be challenging for you to stick to the boundaries that you set due to feelings of guilt or your loved one's response or behavior toward your boundaries. However, it is important that you push past this uncomfortable transition and follow through with the boundaries you set.

When a boundary is crossed, assert yourself and remind your loved one about your previously discussed limits. Do so with kindness and assertiveness, maintaining a balance between respect for their struggle and respect for your needs.

Realize that you have the right to say 'no'. It might feel challenging, especially when you want to help your loved one and alleviate their pain. But respecting your own capacity is essential in ensuring you remain a strong and effective pillar of support.

Understand that setting boundaries does not make you a lesser caregiver. It's an act of courage and authenticity that strengthens the caregiving relationship while preserving your wellbeing. Healthy boundaries ensure you remain emotionally, mentally, and physically equipped to face the challenges and victories on the journey ahead.

These are not walls meant to keep love out, but fences that protect your capacity to love without depleting yourself. As a caregiver, your love and support can work wonders for your loved one. But to continue being the beacon of light they rely on, you must first ensure that your own light isn't dimming.

Practice Empathy and Understanding

Up to this point, a great deal has been discussed about different facets of mental health and navigating relationships in the context of mental illness. However, a fundamental principle that sustains all these steps and strategies is empathy and understanding. As we delve into this section, we'll explore how you can purposefully cultivate these attributes to strengthen your bond with your loved one and support them effectively.

Empathy is often confused with sympathy, yet they offer different perspectives. While sympathy involves feeling sorry for someone else's distress, empathy involves seeking to understand and share that person's feelings. Embodying empathy means not merely recognizing someone's pain but also connecting with it. Empathy allows us to feel with others, not just for them.

Evolving your perspective to focus more on empathy can lead to deeper connections. As you relate with your loved one, consciously acknowledge their feelings and validate their experiences. It can simply involve giving them space to express their feelings–a nod or a comforting phrase such as "that sounds really tough," can go a long way. By acknowledging their feelings, you're communicating that their emotions are real, valid, and important.

It's equally essential to remind yourself that your loved one's experiences are unique. It's often tempting to compare their journey with mental illness to others' or your experiences. This kind of comparative mindset can weaken your ability to empathize; keep in mind that everyone's experience with mental illness is unique and personal.

Understanding the mental illness your loved one is dealing with is also crucial. This doesn't imply that you must know everything, but an informed perspective is always beneficial. To facilitate this understanding, you can read up on the disorder, speak to professionals, or join support groups. Encouraging your loved one to share their experiences can also enhance your comprehension.

While it's important to understand the illness, remember that your loved one is more than their diagnosis. Remember the individual behind the illness-their strengths, interests, goals, and quirks. This focus helps prevent your relationship from becoming one defined solely by the mental illness.

Patience is another key aspect of empathy. Progress is often slow when dealing with mental illness, with good and bad days interspersed. There might be times when your loved one may seem to be taking steps backward despite your efforts. Understand that recovery is a bumpy journey, and it's essential to display patience during these difficult times.

While empathizing, strive to maintain a positive, yet realistic, attitude. Being overly negative can create a tense atmosphere that may hamper communication, while being unrealistically optimistic can seem dismissive of reality. Keep a balanced outlook, with a focus on growth, however small it might be.

Practicing empathy also means respecting your loved one's autonomy. Despite their mental illness, they have the right to make decisions about their lives, including their treatment. By recognizing and respecting their choices, you validate their agency. Convey your concerns, but remember it is ultimately their decision.

To further increase understanding and empathy, try seeing the world through the lens of your loved one. This doesn't mean you have to agree with all their thoughts or perceptions, but it does mean recognizing that their feelings are grounded in their experiences and perspectives. Their fears, anxieties, or frustrations may not seem rational to you, but to them, they're very real. Recognizing this can help you to respond with more empathy.

Communication is key when promoting empathy and understanding. Check your tone, phrasing, and intent. Strive to communicate in a way that's devoid of blame, judgment or criticism. Instead, use "I" statements and express how their actions impact you. This way, you can communicate feelings without making the other person defensive.

As you work on empathy, remember it's a continually evolving process. You might not always get it right, and that's okay. What's important is the conscious effort to understand and connect with your loved one. Prioritize empathy and understanding in all your interactions; over time, this will become second nature.

Don't lose sight of the fundamental goal: Supporting your loved one as they maneuver their path through mental illness. Your empathy and understanding can significantly influence their journey, making them feel heard, validated, and less alone in their struggle.

In the end, empathy and understanding are not just practices; they're a mindset-a lens through which you view and approach the world. And when applied consistently, they can transform your relationship with your loved one, creating an atmosphere of acceptance, respect, and mutual support.

Fostering Mutual Respect and Trust

The journey of supporting a loved one with a mental illness is often broad and complex, but one of the most valuable investments you can make is in cultivating a foundation of mutual respect and trust. This gives strength to the relationship and offers a meaningful space for growth, recovery, and resilience. Let's delve deeper into how we can build this essential dynamic.

Recognition is a powerful tool in building respect. Understanding that mental illness is not a failure, but rather a challenge that anyone can face, can aid in fostering a climate of respect. Especially towards your loved one. Validate their experiences, strive not to judge their actions or feelings, and accept that their reality, though different from yours, is just as real and valid. This isn't to say you have to agree with everything your loved one feels or does, but you can attempt to understand their perspective.

It's pivotal to treat your loved one with dignity, even in times when their behaviors may feel challenging. They are more than their illness, and it's essential to remember that their worth isn't determined by their struggles. Seeing them for who they truly are fosters a deep level of respect and can greatly empower their mental health journey.

Listening is another vital aspect when encouraging respect. It's in these moments of quiet attentiveness where respect is often born. Show interest in their thoughts and feelings, and genuinely seek to understand their point of view. Allow them space to express themselves without interruption or criticism, and respond with empathy and understanding.

Respect can also be developed through consistency in your actions. Follow through on your promises. Making decisions and taking actions that are aligned with what you say fosters authenticity and trust. Trust isn't built overnight, it often comes gradually, brick by brick, through your consistent actions.

Beyond respect, trust is another pillar in building a strong relationship. Building trust takes time, but that investment reaps considerable benefits for both parties involved. Keep in mind, the process of building trust isn't linear; there will be bumps and setbacks along the way. It's how these are navigated that matter most.

Honesty and transparency are the backbone of trust. It's imperative to have open and honest dialogues about mental illness, its impacts, and the journey ahead. This begins by being true to your feelings and sharing them with compassion and sensitivity. Be open about your own shortcomings and vulnerabilities, which can invite your loved one to do the same.

Building trust with a loved one dealing with mental illness also involves preserving their autonomy. Allow them to make decisions for themselves whenever possible, and provide guidance and support when necessary. Their journey to mental health is ultimately theirs to make, and your role is to walk alongside them rather than lead.

Apart from being a mental health supporter, never forget your role as a loved one-a parent, a sibling, a partner, a friend. Shared positive experiences can deepen intimacy and trust. Spending time with one another doing something fun and entertaining can provide a positive impact on your relationship with your loved one that can take you out of the caregiver role and back into the role of friend or family member. This can help your loved one see you as an ally again after a rough patch, it can allow you both time to decompress by having fun, and can strengthen the relationship as a whole. In building trust it is also important to remind your loved one of their strengths and accomplishments, and to encourage and celebrate their victories, no matter how big or small.

One of the most potent ways to establish trust is by ensuring the consistency between your words and actions. Be a person of your word; delivering on promises and commitments can strengthen the bonds of trust over time.

The process of fostering mutual respect and trust with a loved one grappling with mental health issues can be a daunting task. It can be filled with immense challenges, heightened emotions, and a considerable amount of patience. But remember: each step forward, no matter how minuscule, is a step towards a stronger bond and a healthier relationship.

As you journey in fostering mutual respect and trust, it's essential to acknowledge the progress you've made, but also to be patient with the process. Trust and respect are not static milestones, but rather a continuously evolving dynamic that requires constant attention, nurturing and reassessment.

In building this mutual respect and trust, there may be times when you make mistakes or misstep. This is completely normal. These moments can serve as valuable opportunities for growth and learning. It's crucial to take these in stride, apologize when necessary, and persevere through the rough patches together.

Through consistent effort, open communication, and a firm commitment to understanding, it's possible to cultivate mutual respect and trust with a loved one dealing with mental illness. This nourishing environment can contribute to stronger bonds, better mental health outcomes, deeper understanding, and a more fulfilling relationship.

In the following chapter, we'll discuss how to cope during crisis times while keeping this foundation of mutual respect and trust intact, and how the strategies applied here can prove to be vital in those challenging times. As you navigate through these intricate aspects of managing mental health, the ultimate goal remains, supporting loved ones in their journey towards mental wellness with respect, trust, and unconditional positive regard.

Chapter 5 Key Take Aways

1. Setting healthy boundaries is critical to maintaining a balance between caring for your loved one and your personal needs.

2. Practicing empathy includes patience, understanding, respect, and seeing the world through the lens of your loved one.

3. Building trust includes being consistent with your words and actions, being honest and transparent, and having open communication.

Chapter 6:
Coping with Crisis

When dealing with mental illness in a loved one, you'll inevitably find yourself amidst a crisis-a scenario where the person's mental health situation escalates, posing a risk to themselves or those around them. These moments can be terrifying, but it's important to remember that you're not alone, and there are resources available to help. Recognizing the signs of a crisis is your first line of defense. As a caregiver you've gotten intimate with your loved one's behaviors, making you well-equipped to spot changes. Unusual, erratic, or worsening symptoms are often the first clues, so trust your instincts. During emergencies, maintaining your own calm can be a challenge, yet it's crucial. Reach out to professionals-therapists, mental health hotlines, or emergency services, and follow their guidance. Remember that you're not betraying your loved one, rather you're offering them immediate life-saving help. The aftermath can be hard to navigate. There may be feelings of guilt, discomfort, and a variety of other strong emotional responses. However, it's crucial to learn to manage these feelings, without letting them consume you. Open discussions with your loved one and mental healthcare professionals can help you understand and cope with what has happened.

Recognizing Signs of Crisis

The ability to recognize signs of a crisis in individuals with mental illness is a vital aspect of offering them the support they need. While the specifics can be distinctive depending upon the illness and each individual person, there are several universally acknowledged symptoms to be aware of. Let's delve into these signals, so that you can be better equipped to offer your loved one the help they need during crucial periods.

One common sign is a significant, often abrupt, change in behavior. Perhaps your loved one who used to be an active participant in family dinners has started to prefer his own company. Or a friend who was always the life of the party suddenly finds no joy in social gatherings and chooses to stay home instead. Remember, not all behavioral changes are indicative of crisis-they could simply be having a bad day, but behaviors that are sudden, uncharacteristic, and persist over time, could be a cause for concern.

Another sign to watch out for is difficulty in concentration or expression of thoughts. They might struggle to maintain the thread of a conversation, forget what they were saying halfway through a sentence, or display an inability to focus on a task. It might also manifest as disorientation or a feeling of being "lost". Their speech may become disjointed, their thought process seemingly fractured, and their understanding of reality may seem distorted.

Alterations in sleeping or eating patterns often suggesting an impending crisis. Insomnia, hypersomnia, loss of appetite, or overeating, all hint towards emotional turmoil. Any significant and persistent change in how your loved one is sleeping or eating can be a red flag.

A noticeable deterioration in personal grooming can be a sign of crisis, too. If you notice someone who was once particular about their appearance now disregarding it, or their personal hygiene suffering, they might be in a state of mental health crisis.

An individual suffering from a mental health crisis might also start expressing feelings of despair or persistent sadness. They may express feelings of hopelessness, as if caught in a situation that they believe they cannot change or manage. They might feel overwhelmed or, in severe cases, may express a desire to end their life.

Excessive worry or fear is another key indication of a crisis. Your loved one may appear unusually afraid or anxious, and this could extend to something more severe like panic or anxiety attacks. Any kind of unusual exaggeration linked to an irrational fear or situations that seem harmless to others could point towards a crisis.

In some cases, individuals might also exhibit signs of anger or hostility, which could extend to violent behavior. They may disproportionately react to situations that might seem non-threatening or harmless to others, and have a significantly lower tolerance for frustration.

Withdrawal from social interactions is another common sign of crisis. Your loved one may choose to isolate themselves, prefer solitude over the company of others, and exhibit detached behavior. They might decline invitations to gatherings they would normally attend, stop communicating, or have little or no desire for interaction.

It's important to pay attention to any signs of substance abuse, as this could be a means to self-medicate or escape from their struggles. An increase in alcohol or drug consumption, or the inception of substance use, could indicate an underlying crisis. Substance abuse can be especially dangerous, as it often exacerbates mental illness symptoms and could lead to additional health complications.

A mental health crisis can also include signs of psychosis such as auditory or visual hallucinations, irrational fear of harm from others, and delusional thinking. This can be particularly distressing for the individual, and requires immediate attention and care because of the potential risk of harm to themselves or others.

Observing any of the above behavioral changes doesn't inherently mean the individual is in a state of a mental health crisis. However, it suggests that it might be time to reach out and communicate openly with empathy and understanding. It's crucial to remember that any attempts at intervention should be rooted in compassion and the desire to help, rather than criticism or judgment.

The first move when recognizing these signs is encouraging your loved one to seek professional help, if they haven't already. If they have, and they're open about their treatment, you might consider contacting their mental health care provider to discuss these changes or ask to attend their next appointment with them.

Stay patient, supportive, and persistent. Mental health crises are challenging for everyone involved, but knowing the signs and seeking help can make a world of difference. Remember, you're not alone in this journey; there's help available, and there's hope for healing.

Despite all these signs, you know your loved one better than anyone else. If you see changes or behaviors that concern you, don't ignore your instincts. Reach out, show your support, and encourage them to seek the help they might need. Recognition of a crisis is the first step in effectively responding to it.

Responding to Emergencies

The capacity to respond effectively to mental health emergencies can significantly influence the outcome of these precarious situations. These emergencies could range from a suicidal crisis to severe anxiety attacks or extreme bouts of depression. The response should ideally be swift, knowledgeable, and empathetic-aiming to minimize the likelihood of escalation while assuring the person in distress that help is available, and they are not alone.

One of the critical steps in responding to emergencies is understanding that mental health crises are not deliberate or attention-seeking behaviors but rather the symptoms of a brain illness. Just as a person does not choose to have diabetes or cancer, they do not choose to have mental illness. This understanding is the stepping stone to responding empathetically and effectively.

Active listening, a tool explained in chapter three, is paramount in these circumstances. Often, when your loved one is in a crisis, they may feel unheard or misunderstood, heightening their pain and isolation. Active listening can help reassure them that their feelings are important and valid, and they are not alone in their struggle.

When responding to emergencies, it's essential to strike a delicate balance. You should remain calm and composed, but it's equally important to reflect your genuine concern for your loved one's wellbeing. Displaying panic may potentially aggravate the situation, while displaying a lack of concern might intensify their feelings of loneliness and despair.

However, it's also critical to make it clear that mental health crises, especially suicidal ones, are beyond the capabilities of a loved one's care alone. In these situations, involving competent professionals, such as a psychiatrist or a mental health crisis team, is highly advisable. Giving them immediate access to professional help can mean the difference between life and death.

If your loved one is suicidal, never leave them alone. Constant companionship can provide reassurance and safety. Encourage them to contact their mental health provider or a local mental health crisis line. If they won't, it's crucial to do so yourself without hesitating.

Also, do remember to remove any means of suicide, such as firearms, sharp objects, or an excessive amount of medications, immediately and discreetly. This step alone can be life-saving.

It's also crucial not to make any promises of confidentiality, particularly when a loved one's wellbeing, or even life, is at stake. Although trust is critical, it should not trump safety in these critical situations. It's important to explain that you might need to involve others to ensure they get the help they need.

It's crucial to avoid dismissive attitudes during a crisis. Statements like "It's not that bad," "You're overreacting," or "Just relax" can exacerbate feelings of despair. Such attitudes might discourage your loved one from reaching out for help in the future again. Instead, you could say "That sounds really difficult, how are you coping," "What can I do to help," or "I'm sorry you're going through this, I'm here for you if you need me."

In some instances, you may need to consider medical intervention, which could involve hospitalization. This might seem daunting, but remember, it could be critical to ensure their safety in a severe crisis. The experience could also be therapeutic by moving the individual away from the triggering environment and providing the chance for a reset.

Many areas have mobile mental health crisis teams that can respond on-site, which is less traumatic than law enforcement intervention. They can assess the situation, provide short-term crisis resolution, as well as arrange immediate transfer to a hospital if necessary. They can also provide support in arranging aftercare and ongoing treatment following the crisis.

In emergency situations, it's easy to fall into a "crisis mode" where the whole focus becomes the crisis. However, it's essential to continue with regular routines as much as possible. This can provide stability and a sense of normality during an otherwise chaotic time.

Finally, during these critical situations, remember to prioritize your own wellbeing. It can be incredibly hard to see a loved one in severe distress and not let it consume you. Make sure to reach out to your support systems and engage in self-care. A calm, clear, and focused mind is crucial to providing effective aid during a crisis.

Coping with mental health emergencies of a loved one can be an overwhelming experience. However, the knowledge and strategies provided will equip you to respond with empathy and understanding, ensuring the safety and care of your loved one while protecting your emotional wellbeing.

Dealing with the Aftermath of Crisis

The crisis has passed, and you're left standing amidst its aftermath. It's time for recovery for both you and your loved one and to begin the healing process. This part of the journey can be equally daunting. This part may involve managing symptoms, dealing with the emotional toll, making practical arrangements, and seeking the help you might still need.

Fighting a mental health crisis with a loved one can be a profound experience, layered with complex emotions and questions. You might be feeling a contrast of relief and exhaustion, burdened by uncertainty about what's to come. It's normal to feel this way. Please, don't feel guilty about your feelings, they are natural and justified.

You've learned how to recognise signs, respond to emergencies and face the crisis. Now, let's explore how to navigate through this next stage. As challenging as it may seem, taking it one step at a time will help you emerge stronger on the other side.

Encourage your loved one to seek professional help if they haven't already. Therapists, counselors, psychiatrists and other mental health professionals have the necessary training to guide a person through their journey of healing after a crisis. Restarting or adjusting medication might be necessary to help manage symptoms. It might take some time to find the right therapy or medication, but it's essential to be patient and persistent.

Maintain open lines of communication. After a crisis, your loved one may feel embarrassed, ashamed or guilt-ridden. They won't always be ready to talk, but remind them that you're there when they are. When they do open up, ensure you actively listen, showing empathy and understanding.

After the crisis, your loved one may experience recurring symptoms or new ones. Don't stress; this is often part of the recovery process. Maintain communication with your loved one's healthcare providers to keep them updated and to get necessary guidance and support.

Practical arrangements are another cornerstone in managing the aftermath of a crisis. This may include medical appointments, managing time off work or school, arranging for housing, or financial arrangements. Organising these practical aspects can further alleviate stress and aid in recovery.

Use coping strategies, too. Both for you and your loved one. Deep breathing exercises, grounding techniques, self-expression through art or writing, getting enough sleep, eating a balanced diet; each of these plays an integral role in healing after a crisis. Find what works best in your situation, and stick with it.

It's also crucial to involve other family members and friends in the recovery process. Yes, you've been a significant source of support, but it's healthy and often comforting to have others involved as well. They can provide additional emotional support, assist with practical items, or even share with caregiving duties if needed.

Self-care should be high on your priority list. You can't adequately care for someone else if you're not taking care of yourself. Ensure to factor in some time for relaxation and self-care into each day, which can help you handle stress and maintain your wellbeing.

During this time, you might also consider joining a support group for caregivers. This can provide a valuable space to share your experiences, learn from others who have gone through the same things, and gain advice and support.

Be patient. Recovery from a crisis doesn't happen overnight. There will be good days and bad days, forward steps and setbacks. Celebrate the small victories, and remind both yourself and your loved one that each day is a step towards recovery.

While the road to recovery after a crisis can seem long and foggy, remember that you're not alone. With the right tools, strategies, and support, you can navigate through this journey, always keeping hope on the horizon.

Remember, dealing with the aftermath of a crisis isn't about 'fixing' your loved one or striving for perfection. It's about supporting them, step by small step, as they find their way back, while also taking good care of yourself along the way. You've got this. You're more resilient than you might think.

Chapter 6 Key Take Aways

1. Unusual, erratic, or worsening symptoms are often the first clues of a mental health crisis, so trust your instincts.

2. During emergencies, maintaining your own calm is crucial to help your loved one.

3. Reach out to therapists, mental health hotlines, or emergency services; and follow their guidance.

Chapter 7:
Legal and Financial Planning

As you navigate this complex terrain, you're inevitably faced with the daunting yet crucial realms of legal and financial planning. It's essential to understand and respect the legal rights of your loved one suffering from mental illness. Every individual, regardless of their mental health status, has rights that must be honored. This includes the right to refuse treatment, unless they're a viable risk to themselves or others. Understanding these legalities will not only ensure your loved one's dignity but can also influence their recovery and management process by fostering a sense of autonomy and respect. However, conversations around these issues can be difficult, so it's important to approach them with sensitivity, patience, and care. Additionally, preparing financially for long-term care is a cardinal step. This could involve the exploration of insurance options, understanding government benefits, or even setting up a dedicated savings plan. Remember, the goal is not simply about amassing resources, but ensuring that these resources directly facilitate the well-being and comfort of your loved one. Consider seeking professional assistance, legal advisors and financial planners can offer invaluable guidance on making informed decisions that best serve your loved one's needs. The stress and difficulties that come with supporting a loved one with a mental illness are in no way insignificant, and these matters of law and finance can add an additional layer of complexity. But with understanding, careful planning, and the appropriate guidance, you can confidently navigate this path alongside your loved one.

Understand the Legal Rights of the Mentally Ill

Understanding the rights of a loved one with mental illness is an intrinsic part of providing proper care and support. Their legal rights don't only offer protection but also provide a foundation for ensuring proper treatment, dignity, and respect.

The Americans with Disabilities Act (ADA) prohibits discrimination based on disability, which includes mental health conditions. It ensures equal opportunities for individuals with disabilities in employment, state and local government services, public accommodations, commercial facilities, and transportation.

Under the ADA, employers can't fire, demote, or refuse to hire individuals solely based on their mental health condition. They are also obligated to accommodate the needs of employees with mental illness, within reasonable limits. The first step to request an accommodation from an employer is for your loved one to let their supervisor or human resources department know that they need an accommodation at work because of reasons related to a medical condition. A request for an accommodation does not have to be in writing, they can be verbal. For example, a person who experiences hallucinations may need a longer time frame to complete tasks due to being distracted. They can go to their human resources department in person or over the phone stating they need this specific accommodation. However, though having it in writing isn't a requirement, it may be a good idea to have a paper trail in case there is a dispute about whether or when the accommodation was requested. Many employers do have policies surrounding specific paperwork they would like to have when requesting an accommodation. For example, they may request the employee to complete a form or even get a doctor's note. However, this is not required per ADA policy. While an employer cannot ignore the initial request, this request does not necessarily mean that the employer is required to provide the accommodation. Some employers do go through a lengthy process to determine if the employee's medical condition meets the ADA definition of 'disability.' Sometimes, depending on the accommodation requested, an employer may state they are unable to make the specific accommodation requested, however they may be able to make a slightly different accommodation. For example, a person with ADHD may request to work in a private office space to limit distractions. However, if the employer is unable to provide this space due to space limitations they may provide the employee with noise cancelling headphones or a cubicle at the far end of the office away from most of the noise.

Similarly, public services and privately owned public establishments cannot deny service or accommodation to individuals due to their mental health condition. These rights protect individuals in places like restaurants, hotels, theaters, pharmacies, doctors' offices, and many more locations.

In addition to these broad protections, the Health Insurance Portability and Accountability Act (HIPAA) protects the privacy of medical records. HIPAA guards against unauthorized access to health information. This law accords mentally ill individuals control over who gets to access their mental health records. In order to be able to contact your loved one's mental health and medical providers to access any information or health records from them you will need to get written permission from your loved one to do so. Most health providers have their own forms for this that your loved one can fill out.

The Mental Health Parity and Addiction Equity Act (MHPAEA) is another federal law which requires insurers to treat mental health and substance use disorders equitably with physical health issues. This means that insurance plans that cover mental health must offer benefits comparable to those provided for physical health conditions.

Also key to understanding are the rights of mentally ill individuals in crisis situations. The law necessitates certain criteria be met before involuntary hospitalization can be initiated. In general, a person can be hospitalized against their will only if they pose a direct threat to themselves or others, or if they are unable to care for themselves as a result of their mental illness.

However, the laws for involuntary commitment vary by state and it is vital to familiarize yourself with the ones applicable in your location. In most cases in order to have your loved one involuntarily committed you can't simply tell a law enforcement officer or mental health treatment center that your loved one needs to be admitted into a mental health treatment center; you will need to provide proof along with a doctor's written statement and signature corroborating your claims for them to be involuntarily committed. It is also important to remember that being admitted to a psychiatric facility, whether voluntarily or involuntarily, doesn't strip a person of their basic rights. This includes the right to respectful and humane treatment, the right to be informed and involved in their treatment plan, and the right to privacy.

Advocating for a mentally ill loved one also involves understanding their rights in the criminal justice system. This is particularly important because incarceration rates among individuals with mental health problems are disproportionately high. Mentally ill individuals have the right to competent representation, they have the right to remain silent, the right to avoid self-incrimination, and the right to a speedy, fair trial.

A critical element of these legal rights is the right to a fair trial. This includes the fitness to plead, the insanity defense, and post-acquittal hospital orders. One of the biggest concerns in these cases is whether the person is competent to stand trial, meaning they understand the proceedings and can assist in their own defense.

An insanity defense can be raised if the accused could not understand what they were doing, could not distinguish right from wrong due to the severity of their mental illness, or were compelled by their mental illness to commit the act. It's critical to understand that successfully raising an insanity defense is difficult and it's rarely used.

Despite these strong legal protections, the mentally ill often struggle to exercise their rights fully due to stigmatization, misunderstanding, and a lack of resources. Therefore, part of supporting a loved one with mental illness involves advocating for their rights, increasing awareness, and working to eliminate these hurdles.

Understanding the legal rights of the mentally ill empowers caregivers and loved ones to advocate for just treatment, opportunities, and resources. It lies at the heart of ensuring that your loved one receives the respect, care, and treatment they are entitled to.

In the journey to support your loved one with mental illness, understanding their legal rights is a critical aspect. As a supporter, you can use this understanding to become their advocate, ensuring their rights are recognized and respected.

To sum up, it is crucial to always stay informed about potential legal changes or amendments that might affect your loved ones' rights. Remember that no one should suffer discrimination due to mental illness and by equipping yourself with knowledge, you can truly be a pillar of support for your loved one.

Preparing Financially for Long-Term Care

One part of effectively planning for your loved one's future with a mental illness is understanding how to prepare financially for long-term care. We are often ill-prepared for the financial demands that accompany providing long-term care for a mentally ill family member because we do not always understand the full extent of the costs involved.

The financial toll can include not only medication and therapy expenses but also other related costs such as caregiver wages, home modifications, and transportation needs. For this reason, laying out a clear, comprehensive financial plan is a necessary step in preparing for the future.

Begin by fully exploring and understanding the nature of your loved one's mental illness and the potential long-term implications this will have on their ability to work, live independently, and look after themselves. Each mental health condition, just like any other health issue, comes with its unique set of challenges and necessities, and these must be taken into account while laying out your financial strategy.

Next, get a clear idea of the resources at your disposal. This will include assessing personal savings, insurance coverage, and possible government assistance. It's important to understand what services or treatments these resources will cover, as well as how long that coverage will last. Some insurance plans, for example, may limit the number of therapy sessions they'll pay for in a year.

Consulting with a financial planner can be a crucial step in this process. They not only offer guidance on making the most of your resources but also provide knowledge on investing for future needs and entitlement to disability benefits. Additionally, they often understand the landscape of mental health service financing and can guide you towards less known or under-utilized funding sources.

Consider long-term care insurance as a part of your financial plan. Such insurance can help cover the cost of in-home care, assisted living, or residential care facilities, which may become necessities depending on the progression of your loved one's condition.

Unfortunately, long-term care insurance is not universally affordable and may not be an option for everyone. As such, it's important to start planning and saving as early as possible in anticipation of future health costs.

Look at the possibility of setting up a special needs trust. These trusts can provide financial support for your loved one without affecting their eligibility for government assistance programs, which often have strict financial prerequisites. Legal advice can be helpful during this process to ensure that the trust is set up correctly and efficiently.

Apart from financial planning, family members should also consider estate planning, which includes preparing wills, power of attorney, and if possible, detailed instructions on handling financial matters if the primary caregiver can no longer perform their responsibilities due to unforeseen circumstances.

Sadly, many families face financial hardship after the onset of a serious mental illness, and there's no easy solution. However, knowing your resources and options, planning together as a family, and consulting with professionals can go a long way towards easing the financial stress that accompanies long-term mental health care.

Regardless of the specifics of your loved one's situation or the resources at your disposal, the most important thing is to start planning as early as possible. Just as one would prepare for retirement or a child's college education, planning for the long-term care of a loved one with a mental illness is a necessary, proactive component of financial planning.

While this is a tough journey that no one would choose to embark on, it's comforting to remember that you're not alone. Many families are going through the same challenges and have found ways to navigate the financial complexities. Sharing experiences with fellow caregivers and reaching out for help can give you unexpected breakthroughs and strategies.

Indeed, dealing with the financial implications of mental illness can seem overwhelming. But when broken down into manageable pieces, you can take effective steps to lay the foundation for your family's financial security. It's all part of equipping yourself with the necessary tools to provide the best possible care for your family member afflicted with a mental illness.

Remember, it's not just about the money; it's about ensuring stability, providing peace of mind, and above all, guaranteeing quality long-term care for your loved one. Handling the monetary side of things allows you to focus more on what's most important: your loved one's health, well-being, and happiness through it all.

Chapter 7 Key Take Aways

1. Your loved on has the right to refuse treatment unless they are a risk to themselves or others.

2. Preparing financially for long term care includes insurance options, understanding government benefits, and setting up dedicated savings plans to directly facilitate the well-being and comfort of your loved one.

3. Consider seeking assistance from financial planners and legal advisors.

Chapter 8:
Unpacking Self Care for Caregivers

In this crucial journey as a caregiver for a loved one struggling with mental illness, the risk of emotional and physical toll from the consistent demands of this role is very real. Thus, this chapter delves into the aspect of self-care. Think about it: How can you efficiently assist someone else if your own reservoir of strength and resilience is drained? It's not selfish; it's practical. Understanding the depth and breadth of self-care is a prerequisite to crafting and implementing a sustainable self-care plan. This incorporates the essential elements of rest, nutrition, exercise, and mental rejuvenation. Your wellbeing propels your ability to offer the steadfast support that your loved one requires.

Understanding the Importance of Self Care

As a caregiver, you often prioritize the needs of your loved one above your own. However, neglecting your personal needs can lead to mental, emotional and physical exhaustion. This is where the concept of self-care takes on paramount importance. Honoring the need for self-care is not selfish or indulgent; it's necessary for your overall health and vitality, and crucial for you to be an effective caregiver in the long run.

Just like the announcement on an airplane instructs you to put on your own oxygen masks before assisting others, you must apply the same principle when caring for a loved one with a mental illness. Before you can fully support someone else, you need to make sure that you are in a stable, healthy place yourself.

Self-care refers to the mindful actions you take to cater to your emotional, physical, mental, and spiritual well-being. These actions can include anything from getting a good night's sleep, having a healthy diet, meditation, exercise, or even taking time out to read a favorite book or watch a movie. The importance of self-care lies in its ability to bolster your resilience, enabling you to navigate through tough times without succumbing to burnout.

When neglecting self-care, caregivers might find themselves struggling with feelings of resentment, exhaustion, or frustration which can lead to decreased productivity and effectiveness. Appreciating the value of your own needs can help you realize that self-care is an essential part of your caregiving journey.

Recognizing the importance of self-care can also prevent the onset of caregiver burnout. Caregiver burnout is a state of emotional, mental, and physical fatigue caused by the excessive and prolonged stress of caring for others. By incorporating self-care practices into your routines, you gain the strength and endurance required for sustainable caregiving.

Beyond preventing burnout, self-care helps you maintain a healthy sense of self. It's easy to lose sight of your individual identity, dreams, and aspirations when you're investing so much time and energy into caring for a loved one. Taking time for self-care allows you to affirm your individuality, reduce stress, and promote overall well-being.

Understanding the importance of self-care also empowers caregivers to model healthy lifestyle habits for their loved ones. Those dealing with mental health issues often struggle with maintaining proper self-care. When they see their caregivers practicing self-care, it makes the concept more relatable and encourages them to adopt such practices in their own lives.

You also need to realize that caring for a loved one with mental illness can stir up a wide range of challenging emotions. Self-care can play a significant role in managing these feelings. By creating space to process your emotions, you stay connected to yourself amidst all the challenges of caregiving.

Moreover, consider the freedom and peace that comes from knowing you do not have to neglect your own needs in order to tend to someone else's. Understanding the importance of self-care can liberate you from misplaced guilt about attending to your own needs.

In many cases, self-care can improve your relationships as well. When you are not overwhelmed by stress and exhaustion, you can interact with your loved ones in a more positive, compassionate way. Maintaining your emotional health can help you respond to emotional outbursts or difficult behavior in a calm, constructive manner.

Self-care is not a luxury, it's a necessity. It's not an action that can be put off indefinitely, but a commitment that must be integrated into your daily life. By recognizing its importance, you lay the foundation for a healthier, more balanced caregiving journey.

Through self-care, you're reminded that it's okay to take a pause, to breathe and rejuvenate. This vital understanding allows you to fortify yourself and return to your caregiving role refreshed and renewed. Not only does it benefit you, but it also, indirectly, benefits those you care for.

Remember, self-care is a journey, not an endpoint. It evolves over time, reflecting your needs and circumstances, and it should never be marked by judgement. Rather, it's an act of self-affirmation; a declaration that your well-being matters too.

In the upcoming section, we will discuss how to implement a self-care plan. For now, let's digest the critical understanding needed: self-care is neither selfish nor a luxury, it's a fundamental necessity that keeps you equipped to continue your caring journey effectively and sustainably.

Implementing a Self-Care Plan

As the caregiver for a loved one with mental illness, you dedicate a significant amount of your time and energy each day to deliver thoughtful, compassionate care. This act of giving may leave you feeling drained and might sometimes lead you towards burnout. To prevent this, the creation of a self-care plan is an essential aspect of maintaining your own well-being while effectively supporting the person you're caring for.

First and foremost, a self-care plan is not a one-size-fits-all approach. It is not about a strict set of rules, but rather a guide to help you lead a balanced life in all dimensions: physically, mentally, and emotionally. As a caregiver, identifying your personal desires and needs is pivotal in fostering your own self-care habits.

Drafting a self-care plan may seem intimidating initially, but it becomes easier when broken down into smaller tasks. A good starting point can be setting aside time every day for an activity you enjoy. Whether it's reading, writing, meditating, or painting, these soul-replenishing habits can improve your mood and lower your stress levels over time.

Physical health is an absolute non-negotiable when it comes to implementing a self-care plan. Incorporating regular exercise into your daily routine can work wonders for both your physical and mental health. From boosting your mood through the release of endorphins to improving your sense of well-being, the advantages of exercising are manifold. Provided it suits your schedule, you may opt for including activities like yoga, walking, or running into your routine.

When it comes to food, try to base your diet around nutritious meals that will provide the necessary nutrients your body needs to function optimally. Eating mindfully is equally important. This means paying attention to your body's hunger signals and refraining from emotional eating as a result of stress.

Adequate rest, too, forms a critical part of a self-care plan. Depriving yourself of sleep can hamper cognitive functions and mental health, thereby affecting your ability to care for your loved one. Ensure that you're getting enough sleep and cultivate good sleep hygiene habits like maintaining a consistent sleep schedule and creating a calm, dark, and quiet sleeping environment.

Here's something that's often overlooked but can be incredibly therapeutic: laughter. Laughter triggers the release of endorphins and lowers stress hormones. Indulge in activities that make you laugh. This could be through watching a comedy, sharing a light moment with a friend, or even playing with a pet.

Setting healthy boundaries with the person you're caring for is also an essential aspect of self-care. Being clear about what you can and can't do can prevent feelings of despair and protect your mental health. Remember, it's okay to say no when you need to.

Make a conscious effort to cultivate positive relationships apart from the person you're caring for. Balanced relationships can offer tremendous emotional support. Engage with friends and family or even become a part of support groups and communities who understand your journey.

As you develop your self-care plan, remember to value its importance. It's not a selfish act but a vital one. It's the metaphorical oxygen mask that you need to secure for yourself before you can effectively help others. Becoming proactive about your wellbeing can eventually lead to positive changes that reinforce optimal health, increased resilience, and overall happiness.

It's crucial to re-evaluate and modify your self-care plan as per your needs. The process of self-care is about going through trials and errors to understand what works best for you and what doesn't. As paths wind and evolve, so do you and so should your self-care routine.

Caregiving is demanding, and there will be times when you'll falter in sticking to your self-care plan. It's important during these times to not let guilt seep in. Instead, with kindness and patience, bring yourself back to your routine knowing it's for the best.

Remember that your self-care plan is confidential. It's yours to make, modify, and implement. You don't necessarily have to share it with anyone unless it feels right, and imperative to you. Respect your comfort zone and move at your own pace.

At the end of the day, taking care of your own needs isn't about getting away from caregiving. It's about gaining the strength and resilience to continue the journey.

Chapter 8 Key Take Aways

1. Honoring the need for self-care is necessary for your overall health and crucial for you to be an effective caregiver.

2. Self-care activities are the mindful actions that cater to your emotional, physical, mental, and spiritual well-being.

3. It's crucial to re-evaluate and modify your self-care plan based off of your current needs.

Chapter 9:
Resources and Support

Now that we've explored self-care techniques for you as a caregiver, it's vital to have broader discussion about the resources and support networks that can augment your efforts. This chapter provides an overview of the various outside resources that are available such as mental health professionals, clinics, and support groups tailored for caregivers. Additionally, an array of online resources exist that can help improve your understanding of mental health issues, provide advice for managing crises, and offer platforms for you to connect and share experiences with other caregivers. These resources, combined with the skills you've developed from previous chapters, can empower you to provide the most effective care and find solidarity with others navigating similar struggles. This support network and knowledge base aren't just peripheral options, they're active lifelines that can mitigate feelings of isolation and overwhelm, providing your loved one with a more comprehensive scaffolding of care and support.

Mental Health Professionals and Clinics

The world of mental health treatment is filled with a variety of professionals, all of whom bring different skills, perspectives, and approaches to helping your loved one manage their mental illness. Whether you are just beginning to explore treatment options or are looking for ways to amplify an existing treatment plan, it's important to understand the variety of mental health professionals and what they each contribute.

Psychiatrists are medical doctors who specialize in diagnosing, treating, and preventing mental illnesses. They can prescribe medication, provide psychotherapy, and use treatments like electroconvulsive therapy. Often, your loved one's journey towards treatment will begin by meeting with a psychiatrist to establish a diagnosis and initial treatment plan.

Psychologists, on the other hand, are not medical doctors and generally do not prescribe medication. Instead, they focus on providing mental health assessments and talk therapy to help the individual understand and manage their symptoms. They can be instrumental in teaching coping strategies and working through specific challenges or traumas that may be contributing to your loved one's mental health struggles.

Social workers and licensed professional counselors are mental health professionals that hold master's degrees in their respective fields. These experts often deal with the realities of living with mental illness, such as navigating relationships, balancing work and life, managing stress, and providing mental health therapy to process through thoughts, feelings, emotions, and traumas. Many social workers do not offer therapy services, though provide care coordination services instead.

Alongside these professionals, psychiatric nurses play a vital role in mental health care. They have specialized training in mental health and can provide psychotherapy, manage medication, and coordinate care. Psychiatric nurses often work in hospitals, clinics, and other medical environments, so your loved one may encounter them in inpatient settings.

In addition to individuals, a variety of clinics and institutions offer specialized mental health services. Outpatient clinics can provide a place for your loved one to regularly meet with their mental health professionals, receive therapies, and possibly participate in support groups.

For more intensive care, residential treatment centers or psychiatric hospitals can offer round-the-clock support. These environments allow focused, comprehensive treatment and are often used for more severe mental illnesses or during times of crisis. Visiting these facilities can be distressing, but keep in mind these places exist to help your loved one and to give them the care they need.

Day programs, sometimes called partial hospitalization programs, provide intensive therapies and support but allow the individual to return home in the evenings. This can be a beneficial option if your loved one needs intensive support but is not fully ready to return to their usual day-to-day routine.

Teletherapy, or online therapy, has grown increasingly popular, especially with the rise in remote accessibility. This delivery method allows your loved one to participate in therapy sessions from the comfort of their own home. It might be a great option for those who live in remote areas, lack transportation, or possess physical restrictions that make leaving the house challenging.

Aiming for a mix of different treatments can often bring the most success. Your loved one's treatment team might recommend combining psychotherapy, medication management, lifestyle changes, and other therapies. Finding a balance that suits your loved one's unique needs is crucial.

Just as every person is unique, so is every mental illness. Therefore, when you're finding the right health professionals or clinics, remember that what works for one person might not work for another. It's crucial to find mental health care providers who not only connect with your loved one but also understand their specific needs and challenges.

To find a mental health professional or clinic, ask for referrals from your physician, reach out to your local community health services, or seek recommendations from trustworthy sources. This could include individuals who work in the field, or family and friends who've had a positive experience with a mental health professional or clinic.

Remember that it might take some time to find the right fit, so don't get disheartened if it doesn't happen instantly. It's worth taking the time to find the right professional or clinic that can best serve your loved one's needs.

Ultimately, the goal is to connect your loved one with the care they need to manage their mental illness effectively. By understanding the variety of mental health professionals and clinics available, you can better navigate this journey, confident that you're making informed decisions about their care.

Prepare for Care

We have touched on the various resources available, however it can feel very scary to pursue or begin a program without having knowledge on what to expect. In this section we will touch on the general expectation for various mental health resources and services one might utilize. Though, we can't say for certain how exactly a specific treatment will go, as each clinic and provider has their own policies and procedures. However, in this section you will find a general description of what one can expect.

Let us begin with mental health therapy. Each session is typically 45 minutes to an hour in length. Some therapists use the first session to complete paperwork together and some therapists send you paperwork to complete prior to your session and then go over it with you during your first session to ensure everything is completed. The typical paperwork one would be expected to complete for therapy is an insurance information form, Health Insurance Portability and Accountability Act (HIPAA) form, bill of rights or patient rights form, privacy practices form, authorization of release of information (if you want to share your treatment information with anyone else), and the patient history form. The patient history form is typically a very large packet where you will give your therapist your contact information, mental health and medical history, and reasons that brought you to therapy. Adult sessions and child sessions are typically structured very differently. For adults, the first session will include a conversation about the main reasons why you sought therapy (i.e. trauma, loss of a loved one, problems in a relationship, stress management, etc). The therapist will ask you your symptoms (i.e. anxiousness, fatigue, poor concentration and focus, depressed mood). Your therapist might complete an assessment based off of symptoms you describe, however sometimes this is conducted in the second session. There are several different types of assessments, so describing your symptoms in detail can help your therapist choose the correct assessments to conduct in your sessions (i.e. Beck Depression Inventory, Generalized Anxiety Disorder 7 or GAD-7, Wahler Self-Description Inventory, etc). For a child, the first session will include a discussion with the parent about various questions and concerns and then play with the child. It is important with children to include play in therapy sessions as children don't often open up to one on one conversation with a person they just met who is asking very personal questions. So the therapist will include a board game, playing with a doll house, or blocks while asking general questions of the child like if they have pets, who do they live with, do they like school, etc. It may take time for the therapist and child to build a trusting relationship so the first few sessions may not have a lot of sustenance aside from play and building a therapeutic alliance. Once the therapist finds the child trusts the therapist the therapist can then start to ask more intrusive questions.

There are many forms of therapy; cognitive behavior therapy, dialectical behavior therapy, eye movement desensitization therapy, play therapy, exposure therapy, existential therapy, etc. Which therapy type your therapist might use is based on what you are there to see them for and their credentials, as some therapies need further specialized training and certification.

As you continue with therapy and get comfortable with your therapist you will discuss and explore coping skills, root causes to your symptoms and issues, challenge negative ways of thinking, explore improved communication techniques, etc. At the end of each session your therapist may give you homework or a challenge to work on before your next session. Dependent upon your need, you may attend therapy session weekly, bi-weekly, or monthly. Therapy can be conducted in-person at an office or clinic, or virtually via a computer, tablet, or phone. The overall duration of your time in therapy is up to you and your therapist; you may be in therapy for a couple of weeks, a few months, or a year. Your length of time in therapy is up to you and your therapy goals. Unless you are court ordered to be in therapy, you can end therapy at any time, you are not obligated to attend a specific number of sessions. It is also important to mention that it is also okay to switch therapists. If you don't feel a connection with your therapist let them know you are moving on and find another therapist to meet with that you might feel more comfortable with.

Group therapy is slightly different than individual therapy. You will still have similar paperwork to complete, however, group therapy typically has a general theme such as a group for people who have gone through trauma, people struggling with anxiety disorders or mood disorders, etc. In group therapy you will be in a room with around 3-15 people in addition to the therapist running the group. Typically you will sit in a circle or square so everyone can see each other. The therapist will bring up a topic or ice breaker to get people talking and then each person gets a turn to talk. The therapist gives therapeutic advice when advice is needed. The therapist may also act similar to a teacher, standing at a white board teaching the group a new coping skills or giving psychoeducation. There are often homework assignments in group therapy as well.

Support groups are similar to group therapy, but with a number of differences. You will be in a room with 3-15 people, sometimes more. Seating arrangements are often in circles or squares but not always. Most support groups are free, so there isn't any paperwork you have to complete aside from maybe a sign in page. You can walk in without having an appointment for the support group. You can typically bring a friend, family member, or other support to your group with you if needed. The support group will typically begin with a check-in or an around the room. And then the group members lead the group. The monitor is sometimes a therapist but doesn't have to be a licensed therapist. The role of the monitor is to ensure everyone is following the rules (i.e. making sure nobody monopolizes the time, keeping people on task, ensuring everyone is respectful of one another, etc) and to start and end the meeting. The monitor usually stays pretty quiet during support group. They do not give advice or do any teaching or psychoeducation because they are not a licensed therapist. Usually a support group monitor is someone with lived experience or a volunteer.

An intensive outpatient program is a day program that is an alternative to hospitalization but more intensive than weekly therapy sessions. With intensive outpatient you will complete similar paperwork to beginning with a therapist. However, you will attend several days a week for several hours, many cases you will attend three to five days per week, for several seeks. Each day in intensive outpatient programming you can expect to attend individual therapy, group therapy, maybe some family therapy if needed, and various classes, such as anger management class (depending on the program).

When hospitalized for mental health there will be similar paperwork as the other therapy programs listed above, however there will also be a form to complete to list the property you brought with you so that when you leave they make sure you bring that property with you. Most often during intake the patient will be required to take off all of their clothes and stand naked in front of staff to ensure the patient didn't bring in any restricted items. There is typically restrictions on the clothing you wear, often times they make you wear scrubs or a hospital gown. Sometimes they will allow you to wear street clothing, but without any metal, so mainly sweatpants and cotton shirts with no buttons. Usually you don't get to wear shoes, only slippers or sandals. You wont get to bring in anything alcohol or chemical based, such as perfumes, sprays, face cleansers, etc. Some self-care items such as tweezers, certain combs, etc. are restricted. They will keep nail clippers and such items in a lock box and observe you utilize these items for safety. Typically you are required to stay in your wing or unit. You can't go outside without permission or supervision. You will follow a structured schedule, usually including exercise. You will have limited free time. Most of your day is scheduled with group therapies, individual therapies, and activities. Often times they make you come out of your assigned room at a specific time and will lock the door to your room so you can't go in there until bed time. There is often no alone time for safety reasons. Visitors are often restricted for the first couple of weeks. When you are allowed visitors they have to be above the age of 18, so if you have children younger than 18 years old you will not see them while you are hospitalized. You get one phone call per day to a loved one. The visitation and phone calls can be taken away at any time depending on if you are complying with the program and directives. Hospitalization time is different for everyone. Some people are hospitalized for a couple of days, some for several weeks or months. However, most insurance has a set time limit on what they will pay for, so if insurance stops paying and nobody can pay for the patient out of pocket, then the patient is automatically discharged, even if they are not well. If the patient voluntarily checked themselves in then they can decide to end their stay at any time unless they are a harm to themselves or others. But if they were involuntarily committed they can not check out without being discharged by a judge or clinician.

Support Groups for Caregivers

While your primary focus as a caregiver may be to facilitate the wellbeing of your loved one, it is essential to also attend to your personal needs, emotions, and mental health. Engaging in support networks such as special caregiver groups not only empowers you but it can equip you with assorted resources, skills and reassurance that you are not alone.

Support groups for caregivers are meetings of individuals who share similar experiences. They come together to share stories, offer advice, and provide emotional support for one another. Participating in these circles can counteract the feelings of isolation often experienced by caregivers. Additionally, it can provide a safe environment where you can express your feelings without judgment, and build supportive connections with those who genuinely understand the caregiving journey.

The concept of support groups, while straightforward, holds immense impact. The opportunity to connect with others who understand your situation, and can reciprocate advice, understanding, and empathy, is a powerful antidote to the feelings of isolation and overwhelm that caregiving can bring.

These groups tend to have a therapeutic nature where attendees do not merely vent their frustrations. Instead, they seek to learn, grow, and find ways to adapt to their situations while being catalysts of mutual encouragement to one another. The structure of these groups may vary, some may have a professional counselor leading the discussions, while others could be peer-led.

Another advantage of support groups is that they're a treasure trove of practical advice. Participants often share actionable tips and strategies they've discovered along their caregiving journey. These tips may pertain to managing the rigors of caregiving, dealing with mental health crises, or navigating complex medical or legal systems, areas you might struggle with as a caregiver.

In addition to emotional and practical support, these groups often provide a wealth of information about resources available to caregivers, such as, an understanding of the legal rights of the mentally ill, knowledge about the ideal clinics and mental health professionals, tips for self-care, and possible financial help that can prove advantageous through your journey.

Many of these groups also offer educational programs and advocacy opportunities for those passionate about improving the mental health landscape. Besides, some support groups may offer respite care: temporary care for your loved one to provide you with a much-needed break.

Keep in mind that not all support groups are created equal. To find the right group for you, consider factors such as the group's focus, whether the group is facilitated by a professional, and the group's style. You might also want to consider the values, demographics, and format (whether in-person or online).

While considering these factors bear in mind your personal comfort, convenience, and lifestyle needs. For example, if your schedule is full and you're struggling to carve out time for self-care, a virtual support group might be a suitable option that allows you to participate from home during hours convenient to you.

At times when you find a group that doesn't sit well with you, it's perfectly okay to keep searching until you find the right fit. Remember that you're seeking a setting that will provide growth, relief, and rejuvenation, don't settle for less.

Invited speakers, usually professionals in the mental health field, often guest these groups. Their discussions can help provide you with a more advanced understanding of mental illnesses, causes, effects, and treatment options. This knowledge may help you to provide more effective care to your loved one, bridge gaps of misunderstanding, and reduce the mental strain associated with caring for someone with a mental illness.

It's important to embrace the fact that participating in a caregiver support group doesn't mean that you've failed or that you're incapable of handling your duties. In contrast, it's about empowering yourself with emotional resilience, broadening your knowledge, and activating resources that can enhance your caregiving abilities. It's a step towards strength, inclusivity, security, and better mental health—for your loved one and you.

Asking for help or guidance isn't a sign of weakness; it's an act of courage, self-awareness, and strength. Being able to say, "I need to connect with others; I need support and help," validates your journey like nothing else can. You are not only a caregiver, after all, but a human being with full right to wellness and support.

Whatever phase of your caregiving journey you're in, remember that there are groups out there ready to embrace and support you. By engaging with these groups, you're taking care of yourself. In the long run, building connections and actively participating within a supportive community will not only strengthen you but inevitably empower your journey of providing care for your loved ones.

Online Resources for Mental Health

In today's world, the internet provides a vast array of online resources to help support the mental health of individuals and their caregivers. These tools offer a plethora of information, virtual assistance, self-guided therapies, and online communities that can prove invaluable for anyone dealing with mental health issues. They are essential to understand and take full advantage of.

Websites dedicated to mental health education are a crucial source of accurate, reliable, and understandable information. Sites like NAMI (National Alliance on Mental Illness), MentalHealth.gov, and MentalHealthFirstAid.org provide facts on different types of mental health disorders, their symptoms, causes, treatments, and advice on how to support a loved one struggling with such issues.

Another beneficial form of online resource comes in the shape of self-help platforms. These are specially designed websites and applications that guide users through various techniques to manage their mental health. These may include mindfulness apps, cognitive behavior therapy programs, or tools designed to manage stress, anxiety, or depression. Platforms like Headspace or My Possible Self can be beneficial in this regard.

Teletherapy, or online therapy platforms, are also increasingly popular and accessible. They can connect individuals with licensed therapists via video calls, removing the barriers of transport, travel time, and the need to work around a thermostat's office hours. Teletherapy options include Teladoc, Amwell, and many others.

Then there's the benefit of online peer-support communities. Mental health support groups, forums, and social media communities can provide a sense of connection, understanding, and shared experiences. Sites like Mental Health America offers links to various online communities that cater specifically to those impacted by mental health conditions. Other platforms like Reddit, Facebook or Elefriends also host numerous groups where the participants offer mutual support, understanding, and guidance based on their experiences.

Many nonprofit organizations and governmental bodies have online resources available as well. These include the American Psychiatric Association, the Anxiety and Depression Association of America, the National Institute of Mental Health, and others. They offer research, professional guidance, and treatment options, along with resources directed at individuals and caregivers alike.

Crisis hotlines and support networks can also be accessed online. Text-based crisis lines like Crisis Text Line or the Suicide Prevention Lifeline provide immediate, anonymous help in severe situations. There are specific resources too, for different age groups, backgrounds, and experiences, like the Trevor Project for LGBTQ+ youth or Veterans Crisis Line.

Online courses related to mental health can be another tremendous resource. Websites like Coursera or Udemy provide classes on understanding mental health, managing it, and supporting a loved one who's dealing with these issues. They often include certified classes from known universities or organizations, making them a reliable learning platform.

Another facilitator of mental health care online is the availability of medication management tools. These applications can assist your loved ones in keeping track of their medications, ensuring they are taken on time, and in the correct doses. Apps like Medisafe and MyTherapy can provide significant help in medication management.

Online blogs and vlogs can also play an informative and supportive role. Many individuals share their personal journeys of dealing with mental health issues and their viewpoints can provide different perspectives, offering comfort and assurance that you're not alone.

Resources like online inspirational and stress relief applications may prove beneficial as well. These can provide an inspiring quote to start your day, comfort during the hard times, or help you unwind with some calming music or guided relaxation.

Make sure to bookmark, download, or note down online resources you find helpful. Be open to exploring different platforms or resources before settling on what works for you the best. Remember, it's all about stepping stones towards better understanding and management of mental health.

It's crucial to be discerning too. Unfortunately, not all information found online is reliable or accurate. Always verify the source of any information, what credentials they hold, and whether the information is up-to-date. Avoid anyone promising quick fixes or miracle cures. The best sources of counsel come from licensed professionals and recognized organizations within the field of mental health.

Online resources for mental health are diverse, plentiful, and accessible to anyone with Internet access. It's about finding the right ones that cater to your specific needs or those of your loved ones. They are an important aspect of support, providing you with essential tools to not only learn about mental health but to cope with and manage it effectively as well.

<u>Chapter 9 Key Take Aways</u>

1. There are many different types of mental health professionals: psychiatrists, psychologists, therapists, social workers, and psychiatric nurses.

2. There are many different types of support centers for your loved one: day programs, intensive care, outpatient care, residential treatment centers, psychiatric hospitals, telehealth, support groups, and crisis hotlines.

3. There are many different types of supports for caregivers: therapists, support groups, educational programs, online resources, and crisis hotlines.

Conclusion

As we reach the end of our journey together, the essence of caring for a loved one with a mental illness is becoming clear. It's more than communicating effectively or understanding the intricacies of their situation. It's about blending empathy, knowledge, respect, and even the capacity to cope with the unforeseen. The path is rarely linear and often filled with unexpected turns, but the rewards - the deepening bond, the mutual growth, and the nurturing of resilience - are significant.

Understanding mental illness commenced your journey, as knowledge is a powerful weapon. It helps transform your fears and stereotypes into empathy and compassion. By confronting stigma, you can break down harmful barriers, cultivating a conversation marked by understanding and acceptance instead.

Motivating a loved one to seek help is often complex. Love, patience, and gentle persistence play pivotal roles in overcoming resistance and denials. In the realm of communication too, active and non-verbal cues gain prominence, fostering a dialogue echoing with trust and sincerity.

Stepping into the shoes of a caregiver is a profound responsibility. Facilitating medication routines, ensuring appointments, offering emotional support, and even aiding in job security can all be part of this role. Yet, your assistance should not dissolve boundaries. Setting such limits, coupled with empathy, respect, and trust, fortifies your relationships.

Navigating the choppy waters during a crisis can be arduously challenging. But a crisis does not necessarily herald despair. It offers a unique opportunity to re-evaluate, learn, and grow. Recognizing signs, responding efficiently and dealing with the aftermath is a testament to your resilience and commitment.

Mental health struggles often intertwine with legal and financial conundrums. Understanding this reality and being prepared doesn't translate to pessimism; it's about enduring long-term care without being overwhelmed financially.

As a caregiver, you are an invested care provider, a champion, and advocate for your loved one. In this role, you can often forget about caring for yourself. Prioritizing self-care is by no means a selfish act; rather, it encapsulates the adage, "You can't pour from an empty cup." So honoring your needs, implementing a self-care plan becomes equally significant.

Finding resources and support can alleviate some of your burdens, too. Professionals, support groups, and digital resources can all offer unique perspectives and useful advice, fostering a sense of solidarity in this often-challenging journey.

As we conclude, it's important to remember that no two journeys are the same. Your journey may have different troubles and triumphs, and that's okay. What truly matters is the compassionate and dedicated heart with which you engage in this journey. The love, understanding, and steadfast dedication you bring to this role can help your loved one live a healthier, more fulfilling life.

Remember, it's absolutely fine to make mistakes, stumble, even fall. Each stumble is a stepping stone to learning, refining your approach, and becoming a more confident caregiver. So embrace your journey with its ups and downs, for that's the essence of this unique voyage.

The lessons from this guide offer a roadmap, not a fixed itinerary. It is up to you to adapt the knowledge and strategies to fit your unique circumstances and relationship. As a caregiver, you need to adapt, improvise, and grow, continually learning new ways to support your loved one.

Take some time to reflect, to soak in the lessons you have learned, and to embrace the caregiver's journey with renewed understanding, empathy, and courage. Together, you and your loved one, can navigate the challenging yet transformative path that is mental illness care.

This journey isn't an easy one, but it's a worthwhile one. It's a journey that tests your strength, resilience, and compassion. But ultimately, it is also a journey that shapes you into a more empathetic person, a more enduring supporter, a beacon of hope, and a testament of unwavering love.

Every step taken alongside your loved one is not just about helping them-they inevitably help you, too. The shared experiences, the ebbs and flows-they bind you closer, enabling you both to learn and grow. Your strength becomes their strength and vice versa.

To conclude, your strength, compassion, and resilience mark this journey of caring for a loved one with a mental illness. From understanding to advocacy, crisis management to self-care, each chapter of this guide brands an imprint on your journey. So stride forward with confidence, embrace the information, and continue being the remarkable caregiver you are.